About the author

Moira Carpenter had a successful career in marketing, until PMT-related symptoms, beginning in her early thirties, eventually became so severe that, despite contacting top specialists in England and America, she was forced to give up full-time work. After research in alternative medicine, she managed to cure herself completely, and subsequently opened a Premenstrual Tension Centre – the first of its kind in the country – where women could receive advice on overcoming PMT symptoms without resorting to medication.

Also available from Century

The Bristol Diet *Dr Alec Forbes*
A Gentle Way With Cancer *Brenda Kidman*

CURING PMT

The Drug-Free Way

Moira Carpenter

CENTURY PUBLISHING
LONDON

Drawings on pp. 102-3 based on photographs from
Acupressure Techniques by Dr Hans Ewald (Thorsons, 1984)

First published in Great Britain in 1985
by Century Publishing Co. Ltd,
Portland House,
12-13 Greek Street, London W1V 5LE

Reprinted 1985

ISBN 0 7126 0723 4

Photoset by Rowland Photosetting Ltd,
Bury St Edmunds, Suffolk

Printed in Great Britain in 1985 by
The Guernsey Press Co. Ltd, Guernsey, Channel Islands

'The cure of the part should not be attempted without treatment of the whole. No attempt should be made to cure the body without the soul, and if the head and the body are to be healthy you must begin by curing the mind . . . for this is the great error of our day in the treatment of the human body, that physicians first separate the soul from the body.'

Plato, *The Republic*, 382 BC

'I honour physicians not for their services but for themselves. I have known many a good man among them, and most worthy of my affection. I do not attack them, but their art.'

Montaigne (1533–1592), *Autobiography*

Acknowledgements

My thanks go to family and friends who helped and encouraged me on my journey to good health – with a special mention to F.M.

The views and judgements contained in this book are my responsibility, but I would like to thank the following for their assistance and support: the Homoeopathic Development Foundation, Linda Greenbury, Keith Lamont, Victor Perfitt, Howard Thomas, Gail Rebuck, my editor and Darley Anderson, my agent.

Last but not least, my thanks to Joan Gibson and Jean Kirkness for the hours they spent behind their typewriters.

Contents

Introduction   ix

1   Why PMT Occurs   1

2   Hypoglycaemia   11

3   How to Diagnose PMT   15

4   The Role of Nutrition   18

5   Weight Loss can be Easy – When you Know How!   42

6   Vitamins, Minerals and Dietary Supplements   47

7   Homoeopathy and Homoeopathic Remedies   59

8   Herbalism and Herbal Remedies   81

9   Stress and Strain   90

10   Relaxation, Acupressure Techniques and Exercise   96

11   Case Histories   108

12   Useful Contacts   114

13   Summary Charts   120

Reading Material   124

Monthly Charts   125

Index   137

Introduction

'. . . and it all started with custard and raisins.'

'Moira, I'll never forget you sitting in bed eating a huge bowl of custard and raisins late at night. It was a sure sign your period was about to start.' These words were said recently by a friend who shared a flat with me in the early seventies. Although I was unaware of it at the time, this was the first indication of premenstrual tension. Nor could I possibly forecast that ten years later I would be unable to work because of the severity of the symptoms, and that according to medical opinion this situation was unlikely to change until the menopause.

Why am I starting a book on PMT with a detailed account of my own case? Because many of you who are reading it will be feeling desperate, frightened and lonely – and some may even fear mental instability. Hopefully you will read this section before turning to the chapters on remedies, and will find one or more symptoms to which you can relate – this is where hope lies. Just remember as you read my account that I am now completely clear of symptoms after years on drugs. You can look forward to the same result.

The fetish for custard and raisins continued to occur just before each period, but as soon as menstruation started I would revert to my normal eating habits. I had a good job, adequate income, opportunities for plenty of travel and a lively social life; at the start of my thirties life was stabilizing – or so I thought.

I began to notice that 2–3 days prior to each period my breasts would become very sore and heavy. The local doctor prescribed tranquillizers and diuretics for 'the bad days'. I dutifully swallowed the drugs but they constantly refused to work. Empty custard and raisin packets filled the rubbish bin, along with chocolate wrappers and empty crisp bags. I continued to frequent the surgery with monotonous cyclical regularity until it reached the point where I would phone the receptionist, place my monthly order and collect it later in the day. It was a medical take-away. Sore breasts were followed by the first signs of depression. Once again I was back in the surgery, to be referred to the local hospital which in turn prescribed progesterone tablets which did nothing to relieve the symptoms.

By the time I was thirty-five, fatigue had set in and the symptoms were lasting for 7–10 days prior to my periods. I was gaining weight, disliking myself, feeling ugly, crying at the slightest little thing, cancelling social engagements, losing my confidence, taking time off work . . . and I was tired, *very* tired. At thirty-seven, I had a package of symptoms which began two weeks prior to my period and lasted until the second day of menstruation. I left work, since my days off were too numerous to be acceptable. Out of the month there was only one week clear of PMT and menstruating; during this time I would be full of plans and ideas, but there was always an undercurrent of gloom and despair in knowing I would never be able to carry my schemes through. A typical PMT day consisted of rising at 8 am, doing the day's shopping, walking home and by midday returning to bed exhausted.

Often I felt suicidal and eventually made an attempt to end it all with a variety of tranquillizers given by my prescription-happy GP. As the tablets took effect, however, thoughts went to my family and guilt and remorse set in at the anguish I was about to cause. Dressed in night-clothes I drove to the nearest hospital – a car hooted at an intersection – and the next thing I remember was being wheeled down a long corridor by a hospital porter who was saying, 'Don't worry, my dear, you'll be all right.' The hospital report read that the patient appeared very worried and anxious and referral to a therapist was suggested. I kept the first appointment but was still waiting to be seen one hour later so, feeling very ill and despairing that anything could help, I left.

Life had become meaningless and now fear set in about the future. I turned to the Samaritans, a wonderful organization. Many a kind, gentle voice would listen while I talked myself back to sanity . . . until the next time.

Colic pains erupted and often I could only lie on the floor motionless, waiting for the agony to pass. I was physically and mentally at rock bottom. Doctors and hospitals in England had been unable to help, so the next move was to America for three days of tests at a well-known clinic. They could find nothing to account for the colic and ulcer-type pains, but PMT was diagnosed and I left with more tablets. Within ten days I was worse than ever; I felt as though knives were twisting and turning inside my breasts and the fatigue and depression were overwhelming.

Shortly after returning from America, I read a book on PMT by a leading expert and spent many hours checking and double-checking the information against my own experience. I had to wait two months for my first appointment with this doctor, during which time I came off all drugs and tried acupuncture which gave relief, particularly with the stomach pains. Eventually I was seen and – after the results of a blood test were known – the doctor felt sure that I would find relief from progesterone suppositories. Over the next two years the dosage was increased to four suppositories per day from day eleven until the second day of menstruation – a daily intake of 1600 mg of progesterone.

Initially I was delighted – the water retention reduced and the depressions were not so severe – but as time went by my other symptoms became even worse. During the premenstrual phase I would sleep every afternoon and wake up feeling like a lead weight. Tears were never far away, the sugar/carbohydrate cravings hit with a vengeance and my skin came out in a rash. It never occurred to me that I should stop using the suppositories; I assumed that as the suicidal tendencies had gone my continuing problems were totally PMT-related and not the side effects of the drug. Desperation drove me to learn how to inject myself with progesterone; again there was little improvement.

The real bombshell came when doctors confirmed that these symptoms were unlikely to improve until the menopause, and part-time work was suggested. With a recession in full tilt, and now nearing forty, it was obvious that finding a company which would employ me for twelve days each month would be far from easy. I negotiated a bank loan to finance study for a musical qualification, the money being planned to last the year I anticipated it would take to complete the course. PMT quickly put paid to this time schedule – too many afternoons were spent sleeping.

You often hear the phrase, 'things can only get better', and this was true for me when a friend mentioned she had seen an article on homoeopathy and PMT. I tracked down the periodical and was soon on my way to see a homoeopath on the South Coast who had been highly recommended. Although frightened to stop taking the suppositories, I did in fact decide to throw them away and within days was feeling slightly better. It would be wrong to pretend that all was plain sailing, however. Migraine-type headaches plagued me for four weeks and severe depression brought tears and the old feelings of fear, but underneath I felt a glimmer of hope. My period – which had been black in colour, scanty and delayed – reverted to normal and energy slowly returned. I visited companies which dealt in drug-free remedies, tried many of them for my remaining symptoms and started to document the results. I had slightly modified my diet, but was still finding sugar and carbohydrate cravings difficult to control.

By this time I was reading everything I could lay my hands on in order to find a solution to the fatigue which was present off and on throughout the month. After reading a book on low blood sugar (hypoglycaemia), I went for tests and the results showed a pre-diabetic state. Further examination by a doctor of acupuncture revealed that not only were my hormones underactive and depleted but also my glands, adrenals and thyroid. Acupuncture became a regular feature of my life, along with various dietary supplements and a complete revision of my diet. Within three months I was feeling like a new woman, with no PMT symptoms and an initial weight loss of fourteen pounds.

I was so relieved that I offered to help a small group of friends who also had PMT. I quickly found out that my own cure was not unique – the results were startling. Some complete cures occurred in the first month and even for those who took longer there was usually improvement in the first cycle. What was impressive was that nobody went through the long eleven months it had taken me to get back on the road to good health.

It was obvious that this kind of help should be made available on a larger scale, so I searched for small premises in Surrey and started up the first Premenstrual Centre of its type in the country.

In Chapter 11 you will find a number of case histories of women seen at the Centre, which will help you to understand the importance of nutrition and appreciate that many remedies or combination of treatments can cure your symptoms. These cases also show quite clearly that we are all individuals who respond in different ways. Armed with this knowledge, you can start a journey towards a life which need not be ruined by a variety of debilitating symptoms.

CHAPTER ONE

Why PMT Occurs

Far too many women today are complaining of a wide variety of symptoms which can occur anything up to two weeks prior to menstruation. The range is diverse and includes sore breasts, weight gain, sugar and carbohydrate cravings, depression, fatigue, mood changes and headaches. Normally these symptoms reduce dramatically within forty-eight hours of the onset of menstruation. Within the medical profession there are as many conflicting views on what causes them as there are on what treatments to give. Nobody is even certain of the number of women affected by the symptoms, as estimates swing from 40% to 80%.

Added to all this confusion is another problem. None of the drugs being prescribed have been properly tested for long-term evaluation and no doctor has the right to tell a patient that there will be no long-term effects. The truth is that no one knows. Furthermore PMT has been called an 'unrecognized illness' and a 'syndrome'. These descriptions make it something that has to be treated by doctors, which too often means that drugs are prescribed without any real investigation, and with no consideration of the woman as a whole person.

To say that PMT is an illness is worrying on a number of counts. It divides women from women. There are a number of cyclical changes which take place during the lifetime of a woman, and we do not consider 40% to 80% of all pregnant and menopausal women to be ill! The medical profession is attempting to show that during their reproductive years vast numbers of women are ruled by their hormones, thus making them a trial and tribulation to their families and a burden to industry. It is my opinion that a great deal of suffering goes on today because women are misinformed – or at best inadequately informed – on all the contributory causes of the numerous symptoms which can make life a misery.

Far too many of us have been brought up to believe that the doctor will give us a pill to make us better, whereas in the case of PMT there is much that we can all do to help ourselves. Our health and well-being are matters of personal responsibility, and we need to rethink our own attitudes. For instance, we read constantly, 'How to cure PMT'; why do we never read, 'How to *prevent* PMT'? In 1985 the medical profession is still predominantly male, and I am quite certain that if men found they had a range of uncomfortable symptoms month after month, year after year, the research laboratories would be jam-packed!!

All the time we speak about how rotten we feel – what about the good things which can happen during the latter half of the cycle, such as increased creativity and energy? How many women, just before their period, go on a whirlwind tour of cleaning the house, catch up on correspondence or empty the 'In Tray' at work? Instead we read and hear about the negative aspects, go around with a label 'PMT sufferer', accept our lot in life and feel we have nowhere to turn for help. No wonder we are ill!

We must understand the workings of our own bodies and learn as much as possible about everything which can cause PMT, realizing that there is still a great deal to be done in this particular area of women's health.

The Monthly Cycle

Most of us have a period on a monthly basis; the cycle can be anything from 24 to 37 days. If your period arrives regularly on a 31-day cycle, then this is what is normal for you, so don't be concerned about textbook 28-day cycles. Menstruation is simply the process of shedding the lining of the uterus (the endometrium) which increases in thickness throughout the month to prepare for conception (a fertilized egg). If pregnancy does not occur the lining becomes obsolete, is shed, and your period takes place.

The monthly cycle is a very finely balanced feedback system, managed by the hypothalmus – a glandular centre about the size of a greengage located in the brain. Its function is to receive and send out nerve signals to other parts of the brain, regulating functions such as sleep patterns, hunger, thirst and menstruation. It is highly sensitive to stress and illness which can cause hiccups in the signals to the pituitary gland, resulting in possible irregularities in the menstrual cycle.

The pituitary gland, also centred in the brain, produces hormones required to stimulate all the other glands in the body. It also produces the two hormones which stimulate the menstrual cycle:

Follicle stimulating hormone (FSH) which produces the hormone oestrogen. Oestrogen prepares the womb lining for the arrival of the egg.

Lutenising hormone (LH) which is released into the bloodstream. It travels to the ovaries, (sited in the pelvic region) with one objective – to ripen a follicle, causing it to break open and release an egg. The egg travels to the fallopian tube, where it remains for 12–36 hours so that it can be fertilized.

Ovulation has now taken place.

The scar left behind the egg is the corpus luteum, which produces more oestrogen as well as another hormone, progesterone.

Oestrogen rebuilds the womb lining after menstruation.

Progesterone thickens the womb lining to receive a fertilized egg.

When an egg is not fertilized the corpus luteum becomes smaller and dies away and the progesterone levels fall. A few days later, the unfertilized egg is shed and your period starts.

It is clear that hormone levels do alter throughout the cycle, and for many years it was considered that the drop in progesterone levels during the latter half of the cycle was responsible for PMT-related symptoms. Dr Katharina Dalton, a London physician, wrote the first medical paper on the subject to appear in British medical literature and also a number of books including, in 1979 *Once a Month*. Dr Dalton's opinion was that the lowering of progesterone in the latter half of the cycle was responsible for the many symptoms occurring during this time. Her solution was

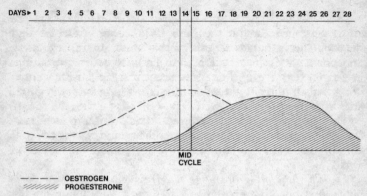

DAYS▶ 1 2 3 4 5 6 7 8 9 10 11 12 13 | 14 | 15 16 17 18 19 20 21 22 23 24 25 26 27 28

MID
CYCLE

— — — — OESTROGEN
/////// PROGESTERONE

Figure 1: Oestrogen and Progesterone Levels Throughout The Cycle When Conception Has Not Taken Place

to prescribe either progesterone suppositories or progesterone injections which increase the level of this hormone in the blood. However, clinical research has shown that 60–70% of PMT sufferers may have progesterone levels within the normal range, therefore progesterone therapy is not the answer for the majority of women. What about women who do have low progesterone levels? I had a blood test, known as a radioimmunoassay, which showed a low level of progesterone, yet suppositories and injections did not work for me. I have met many others who have tried progesterone suppositories, and have yet to find one who was 100% happy with the result; it appears that for most women these merely take the edge off the symptoms.

Dr Dalton's work has been controversial on two counts. First, an American doctor, Penny Wise Budoff, says in her book *No More Menstrual Cramps and Other Good News* that the general impression given by Dr Dalton is that women are unstable. I agree. The 'fickleness' of women has been used over the years as an excuse to keep them 'in their place'. In her book *Once a Month*, she suggests that women's 'temperamental changes' can be related to the changing balance of their menstrual hormones.

Dr Dalton's solution is to help the individual woman by administering drugs, with no consideration whatsoever of other important factors which can contribute to PMT.

Second, other researchers have been unable to duplicate Dr Dalton's experiments and findings. Work done by Dr Gwyneth Sampson* in Sheffield suggested that there was no difference between progesterone and placebo. The placebo always rated as more effective, though not significantly so, and whether progesterone or placebo was administered 60% of women reported improvement in the first cycle. This falls in line with the success rates reported on other treatments. These findings pose some interesting questions. How much of the improvement is due to—

A positive attitude on the part of the woman?
Receiving care and attention?
Having an outlet to discuss the subject?

There is a third hormone secreted by the pituitary gland known as prolactin, which can alter the amounts of oestrogen and progesterone secreted throughout the month. Prolactin stimulates breast milk, but is also produced during the menstrual phase, when too high a level causes breast enlargement and tenderness. Again, most women have normal levels of prolactin. What is interesting in recent research is the finding that deficiency of essential fatty acids (EFAs) can cause the same symptoms as a raised prolactin level.

Essential fatty acids (EFAs) are like vitamins; they cannot be made in the body, but have to come from food. There is another name for them – *polyunsaturates*, of which you will have heard. The most important EFA is *linoleic acid*. So when you read anything which encourages the intake of polyunsaturated fats – think of linoleic acid. In itself this acid is useless unless it can be activated by the body to become *gammalinolenic acid* (GLA), and here comes the problem – there are a number of factors which block GLA, making dietary linoleic acid practically useless:

1 A diet rich in saturated (animal) fats.
2 A diet rich in processed oils which contain *trans-linoleic* fatty acids. These trans-linoleic acids cannot be made into GLA and they prevent the formation of GLA from natural linoleic acid.

---

*Gwyneth A. Sampson, 'Premenstrual Syndrome: A double blind controlled trial of Progesterone and Placebo.' *British Journal of Psychiatry* (1979), pp. 209–15.

(Processed oils are present in such foods as margarine, cooking fats, crisps, chips, bread, cakes, biscuits etc.)
3 Moderate to high consumption of alcohol. (Roughly 20% of the adult population consume enough alcohol to reduce GLA formation.)
4 Diabetes.
5 Ageing.
6 Lack of zinc, magnesium and Vitamin B6.
7 Viral infections, radiation and cancer.

Natural linoleic acid comes from foods such as safflower oil, sunflower seed oil, corn oil, liver, lean meat, legumes, green vegetables, shellfish and linseeds. It comes in two forms:

1 *Cis-linoleic acid*, which is biologically active.
2 *Trans-linoleic acid*, which is biologically inactive, reacts in the body like saturated fats and actually causes deficiencies of EFAs.

Most vegetable oils contain both cis- and trans-linoleic acid. Figure 2 shows the oils which contain a higher proportion of cis- to trans-linoleic acid. You will note that Evening Primrose oil is similar to safflower oil containing 72% of cis-linoleic acid. The unique quality of Evening Primrose oil is that it contains 9%, by weight, of GLA. The only other known source of GLA is human breast milk.

Most of the GLA in the body then goes on to be converted to another substance, dihomo-gammalinolenic acid (DGLA), which in turn converts to a number of compounds, one of which is prostaglandin (PG)EI.

Figure 3 shows the various stages cis-linoleic acid has to take in order to be converted to prostaglandin. If you have any of the deficiencies listed in stage 1, this is where Evening Primrose oil overrides any shortfall and the path to stage 3 is unimpaired. Evening Primrose oil comes in capsule form with Vitamin E added to stabilize the oil. Vitamin E is an antioxidant without which peroxidation can take place.

In 1981 St Thomas' Hospital conducted a study, treating 65 women suffering from severe PMT with Efamol (Evening Primrose oil). The important factor with all the women chosen was

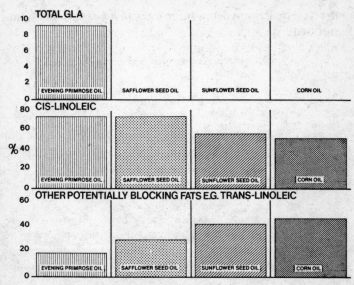

Figure 2: The Linoleic Acid Content of Oils

that they had tried all types of drugs, hormones, tranquillizers etc. and none had worked. After treatment with Efamol the results were as follows:

61% complete relief
23% partial
15% no change

Breast discomfort responded particularly well, with a 72% improvement.

I have already mentioned that the end of the road is the conversion of cis-linoleic acid to prostaglandin E1. Prostaglandins will become well-known over the next few years, since much research is currently being carried out to understand more clearly how they work in the body. They are substances which are produced second by second and which help to maintain the integrity of all cells and organisms in the body. Figure 4 shows how prostaglandins work in the body. Research has produced some very good news for the

Figure 3: The Bumpy Metabolic Road Of Cis-linoleic Acid (Simplified)

Step 1: cis-linoleic acid

↓

enzyme delta-6-desaturase
needed to get to step 2

|

helped by:
zinc, magnesium, Vitamin B6, biotin

|

Blocked by trans fatty acids
Blocked by saturated fats
Blocked by cholesterol
Blocked by too little zinc
Blocked by too little insulin
Blocked by too much alcohol
Blocked by ageing
Blocked by certain viruses
Blocked by chemical carcinogens
Blocked by ionizing radiation

↓

Step 2: gammalinolenic acid
(Evening Primrose oil starts here)

↓

Step 3: dihomo-gammalinolenic acid

|

helped by:
Vitamin C, Vitamin B3

↓

Step 4: prostaglandin E1

Figure 4: How Prostaglandin E1 Works In The Body

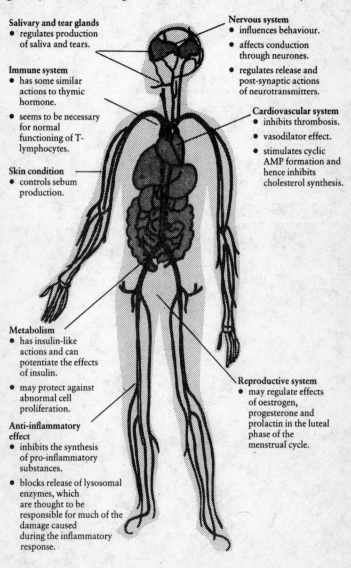

Salivary and tear glands
- regulates production of saliva and tears.

Immune system
- has some similar actions to thymic hormone.
- seems to be necessary for normal functioning of T-lymphocytes.

Skin condition
- controls sebum production.

Metabolism
- has insulin-like actions and can potentiate the effects of insulin.
- may protect against abnormal cell proliferation.

Anti-inflammatory effect
- inhibits the synthesis of pro-inflammatory substances.
- blocks release of lysosomal enzymes, which are thought to be responsible for much of the damage caused during the inflammatory response.

Nervous system
- influences behaviour.
- affects conduction through neurones.
- regulates release and post-synaptic actions of neurotransmitters.

Cardiovascular system
- inhibits thrombosis.
- vasodilator effect.
- stimulates cyclic AMP formation and hence inhibits cholesterol synthesis.

Reproductive system
- may regulate effects of oestrogen, progesterone and prolactin in the luteal phase of the menstrual cycle.

PMT scene – prostaglandin E1 seems to regulate the effects of oestrogen, progesterone and prolactin in the second half of the cycle.

The conclusion must be that a poor diet, abundant in refined and processed foods, plays a significant part in causing PMT symptoms.

CHAPTER TWO

Hypoglycaemia

Hypoglycaemia (low blood sugar) was officially discovered in 1924 by an American, Dr Seale Harris, but the medical profession insist it is a rare disease and a medical condition invented by health food fanatics! There is even controversy as to whether a six-hour glucose tolerance test is a conclusive method of diagnosing hypoglycaemia, or if assessments of the patient's history and symptoms are more reliable. Through all these differences of opinion emerges a clear message – too often the symptoms of hypoglycaemia are mis-diagnosed and put down to stress, neurosis and PMT! Here is a list of symptoms produced by low blood sugar; I have selected only those relating to PMT:

Fatigue	Headaches
Irritability	Food cravings
Overweight	Blurred vision
Joint pain	Lack of sex drive
Anxiety	Depression
Forgetfulness	Lack of concentration
Suicidal tendencies	

Glucose is an important substance in that it provides ready energy for all the tissues in the body.

Hormonal changes before and during menstruation alter blood sugar levels and it is quite possible for women to have symptoms of low blood sugar with a normal level of sugar in the blood. The condition is not always easy to diagnose and to treat hypoglycaemia without professional help is extremely unwise. Moreover, low blood sugar symptoms can also be indications of many serious diseases. Since one of the symptoms of hypoglycaemia is premenstrual tension, I feel it is essential to ensure that women are not diagnosed as having PMT when in fact part if not the whole cause is low blood sugar. It is the lowering of blood glucose – and therefore the reduction of glucose to the nervous system – that leads to the symptoms listed. When glucose levels normalize, all the symptoms rapidly disappear.

The adult brain accounts for 2% of total body weight, yet in terms of glucose requirement it demands 20–25% of available glucose. Under normal circumstances this supply would last about fifteen minutes. A drop in the blood sugar level then hits the circulatory system and the glandular system, in turn affecting the pituitary gland which influences the thyroid and adrenal glands. Inadequate supply of blood sugar to the brain can cause psychological changes, the most common being depression, anxiety and mental confusion. The most common type of hypoglycaemia is reactive hypoglycaemia, the other form being organic hypoglycaemia. In the former, the fasting level of glucose (i.e. the level of glucose in the blood when food has not been taken for several hours) is either normal or a little above, with the body over-reacting to glucose by producing an excess of insulin and causing a drop in blood glucose. The symptoms alter according to the type of food, time of day etc. Organic hypoglycaemia shows a low fasting level of glucose and the symptoms are continuous.

There are various regulatory processes which control the production of glucose and the most important is the hormone insulin. A diet high in sugar fills the blood with glucose it cannot use and causes an over-reaction of insulin; over a period of time the body produces more and more of this hormone, until eventually a slight increase in blood glucose brings with it a high increase of blood insulin. This makes the glands produce adrenalin and cortisone which in turn releases stored glucose, causing even more stress symptoms; the body is then on a merry-go-round – but not so 'merry' for the person concerned!

If untreated, hypoglycaemia can lead to diabetes and although these are two opposite conditions the diets for both are similar. With hypoglycaemia, sugar is avoided in order to allow the pancreas to reduce and insulin output to revert to normal. The diabetic also avoids sugar, as insulin is not being produced in sufficient quantity to convert, transport and utilize the sugar.

If you suspect you have hypoglycaemia, you can be referred to a hospital which will do a fasting blood sugar test; this involves fasting overnight, having a blood sample taken, eating a meal, and then giving more blood samples every fifteen minutes over a two-hour period. I went to a complementary medicine clinic which specializes in low blood sugar, as they considered the symptoms existing *after* two hours to be of primary importance – the NHS only carries out tests for two hours. Reactive hypoglycaemia can only be diagnosed by a six-hour glucose tolerance test.

Members of the medical profession are trained and orientated to the diagnosis and treatment of people with disease, therefore they have concentrated on organic hypoglycaemia which is relatively uncommon. Reactive hypoglycaemia, which is fairly common and probably becoming more so due to the processed and refined foods we eat, is not recognized by orthodox medicine as being clinically significant. The National Health Service is very effective in dealing with major health disorders, but its resources cannot even cope with providing adequate supplies of vital equipment such as kidney machines. Dealing with individual cases showing a slight departure from genuine health takes a low priority, so understandably you may find it difficult to obtain a diagnosis of hypoglycaemia through the established channels.

In most books dealing with PMT low blood sugar is mentioned, yet no serious research has been done on blood sugar levels during the menstrual cycle. Many areas of PMT need examining and in view of the numbers of women involved, this subject should be put high on the list of research programmes. Over the years orthodox medicine has become specialized and compartmentalized. Until doctors begin to look at the implications of diet and stress, stop treating the disease and start treating the person, more and more of us will turn to the 'alternative' approach; while this treatment might be less analytical and scientific, at the present time it is certainly more profound.

This is my reason for writing this book. From now on you are in charge of your own progress and I feel sure you will get a kick out of managing your symptoms, charting your improvement and learning that the natural approach can work and that PMT does not have to be a problem.

CHAPTER THREE

How to Diagnose PMT

For most women PMT symptoms begin anything up to two weeks prior to the onset of their period and normally subside within the first forty-eight hours of menstruation. Over one hundred symptoms have been recorded, but the most common can be classed under the following headings:

TYPE 1 Depression	TYPE 2 Tension
Confusion Lack of concentration Clumsiness	Irritability Aggression Mood changes Anxiety
TYPE 3 Water retention	TYPE 4 Food cravings
Sore breasts Weight gain Bloatedness	Sugar and carbohydrate cravings Headaches Fatigue

It is not uncommon for women to list up to fifteen symptoms which occur regularly every month. This can have a devastating effect on their physical and mental states as well as on their lifestyles. Although exceptionally severe PMT can lead to suicide attempts and extremes of behaviour such as crime and alcoholism, for most women it means anything from mild to severe physical and mental changes. Untreated, this constant strain on the system can lead to other medical problems, so careful diagnosis is of paramount importance. It is equally important that you should be completely honest with yourself. You may well find that your main symptoms appear in the latter half of the month, but that certain symptoms may also crop up at random throughout the month. These should not be ignored, but the cause found. Are they, for example, related to diet or stressful conditions? If in any doubt, seek professional help.

ulcer pains (handwritten marginal note)

Remember: you are susceptible to PMT symptoms if:

- you are in your thirties or forties
- you eat a 'westernized' diet of refined foods
- you are unable to tolerate birth control pills – or they produce side effects
- you gain weight easily
- you have children
- you combine a sedentary lifestyle with little exercise
- you have a stressful lifestyle.

Start by filling in the monthly charts (see pages 125–35), which will show any PMT patterns. (Normally, women with PMT have at least one week free of symptoms.) When you have completed two charts you should be able to tell which symptoms are causing the most inconvenience.

The back of the charts can be used to note down your progress. It is a good idea to record the changes you have made in your nutrition and any vitamin or dietary supplements taken. The same goes for herbal and homoeopathic remedies of course.

In general you should follow these guidelines:

1 Make the necessary nutritional adjustments, noting the major changes you are making, i.e. no coffee, no salt, more fresh fruit and vegetables, reduction in fats, increase in fibre.

2 Note down any vitamin/dietary supplements, herbal or homoeopathic remedies, with strengths and doses taken per day.

It is not advisable to take herbal and homoeopathic remedies together. However, a herbal or homoeopathic remedy can be taken in conjunction with vitamin and dietary supplements. If you have not yet found out which treatments work best for you, though, it is best to try out supplements separately from remedies.

In Chapter 13 you will find master charts listing the symptoms by 'types' and collating the information contained throughout the chapters. This will give you an overall picture of how best to handle your own symptoms.

Continue to document the results carefully by using the charts, as this is the best way to analyse your progress. Should you decide you need professional help, there is detailed information on where to turn in Chapter 12.

CHAPTER FOUR

The Role of Nutrition

The following charts should be filled in before you read the rest of this chapter, as the results will help you to evaluate where change is needed. Chart 1 is a list of foods which should be avoided or significantly reduced, as they can worsen PMT symptoms. Chart 2 lists foods which are nutritionally beneficial and can prevent as well as relieve many of the symptoms.

If you find that you tick a considerable number of the foods listed in Chart 1, you can be fairly certain that your eating habits are contributing to PMT.

Chart 1: Foods That Can Cause PMT Symptoms

(Tick the number of times you eat the foods listed)

FOODS	ONCE A WEEK	TWICE A WEEK	DAILY
Alcohol	✔		
Bouillon-type drinks			
Coffee			
Soft drinks			
Tea			✔
Biscuits			✔
Cakes			
Chocolate		✔	

FOODS	ONCE A WEEK	TWICE A WEEK	DAILY
Honey			
Jam		✓	
Sugar			
Sweets		✓	
Pastry/Pies			
White bread rolls			✓
White flour			
White pastas	✓		⬤
White rice	✓		
Bacon	✓		
Beef	✓		
Lamb	✓		
Mince	✓		
Pork			
Sausages			
Butter			
Cream			
Eggs	✓		
Fried foods	✓		
Full fat cheese	✓		
Full fat milk	✓		
Lard			
Margarine			
Olive oil	✓		
Processed vegetable oils	✓		
Commercial mayonnaise			
Commercial sauces	✓		
Crisps	✓		
Hot spices			
Salt			
Salted nuts			

FOODS	ONCE A WEEK	TWICE A WEEK	DAILY
Savoury spreads			
Stock cubes		✓	
Take-away meals			
Tinned foods	✓		

Chart 2: Foods That Can Reduce PMT Symptoms

(Tick the number of times you eat the foods listed)

FOODS	ONCE A WEEK	TWICE A WEEK	DAILY
Coffee substitutes			
Decaffeinated coffee			
Fruit Juices (unsweetened)			✓
Herb teas			
Mineral water			
Brown rice			
Wholemeal bread/rolls			
Wholemeal flour			
Wholemeal pastas			
Wholemeal pastry			
Chicken	✓		
Fish	✓		
Cold-pressed: Corn oil			
Safflower oil		✓	
Sunflower oil			
Low-fat cheese			
Low-fat yoghurt			
Skimmed milk		✓	

FOODS	ONCE A WEEK	TWICE A WEEK	DAILY
Almonds (raw unsalted)			
Brazil nuts (raw unsalted)			
Hazelnuts (raw unsalted)			
Peanuts (raw unsalted)			
Pumpkin seeds			
Sesame seeds			
Sunflower seeds			
Apricots (dried)			
Dates (dried)			
Figs (dried)			
Peaches (dried)			
Prunes (raw)			
Raisins			
Sultanas			
Apples			✓
Blackberries			
Blackcurrants			
Lemons			
Oranges		✓	
Passion fruit			
Raspberries			
Alfalfa			
Beetroot			
Broccoli	✓		
Brussels sprouts	✓		
Butter beans			
Cabbage	✓		
Carrots	✓		
Cauliflower	✓		

FOODS	ONCE A WEEK	TWICE A WEEK	DAILY
Celeriac			
Chick peas			
Cucumber			
Dried peas			
Fenugreek			
French beans			
Garlic	✔		
Horseradish			
Kidney beans (red)			
Lentils	✔		
Mung beans			
Mushrooms			
Oatmeal	✔		
Onions			
Pearl barley	✔		
Peas			
Potatoes (baked)	✔		
Runner beans			
Spinach			
Spring greens			
Sweetcorn			
Tomatoes	✔		
Watercress			

Throughout this century a great deal has been discovered about the chemical changes which take place in the body once food has been consumed, and we are learning that disease can be prevented and cured by correct nutrition. Pharmaceutical companies, medical schools and universities throughout the world are researching nutrition, all with one aim in view – to get people well, or better still to *prevent* people *becoming* ill. Obviously much is still unknown at the present time, but with the information at hand there is more than adequate proof that we must reassess what goes into our bodies. Nutrition is about building and maintaining good health; provided irreparable damage has not been done healthwise, correct nutrition can put the body back on the road to working correctly and then keep it on course. Nutrition is a science and a full-time speciality, so it is hardly surprising that many doctors are not equipped to give out much more than basic information, with many of the diets years behind scientific research.

The food industry is far from blameless with regard to the nation's ill-health. Products are inadequately labelled. Food is refined and overheated to the point where vital nutrients and vitamins are destroyed and have to be replaced in artificial form. Moreover preservatives, additives, stabilizers and colourings are added – all of which are artificial aids to tempt the senses and prolong shelf life. Until we refuse to purchase this kind of food, the manufacturers will continue to make millions by selling items which at best have little nutritional value and at worst are detrimental to our health.

Change can only begin when shoppers refuse to buy such products. By continually filling the supermarket trolley with refined and convenience foods, we are creating a demand which manufacturers are only too happy to supply. To instigate change we need to have a knowledge and understanding of the body's nutritional requirements, and during the last few years many books have been published to help us in this respect. Any change is slow, so for many years to come temptation will surround food shoppers, but as processed food is bypassed and fresh produce bought in its place, so alteration in the country's eating habits will begin. It is not without reason that most towns have wholefood shops. For the most part these are catering to the enlightened, but if manufacturers can be persuaded to bulk produce health products, hopefully prices will drop. Competition is healthy!

The enormous increase in the consumption of convenience foods over recent years has been accompanied by a decrease in the intake of natural foods. In its wake has been an alarming rise of many diseases such as heart disease, cancer, arthritis, hypogly-caemia and diabetes. For example, recent research has shown that too high an intake of saturated fats can cause painful swollen joints, lethargy, irritability, mood changes and infertility. As shown in Chapter 2, the symptoms of hypoglycaemia – which is caused by too high an intake of carbohydrates and products containing sugar – include headaches, food cravings, irritability, fatigue, depression and *premenstrual tension*!

Although this chapter is perhaps one of the most important in the book, it is well worth remembering that nutrition can only restore health when nutrients are missing and their absence is contributing to poor health. Good nutrition can help in coping with emotional sickness, but it will not remedy the root causes, such as feelings of unworthiness, rejection or loneliness; these aspects will be dealt with in a later chapter.

Taking into account all the knowledge we have to date on foods and their effect on health, we cannot isolate PMT and ignore the fact that for most women a change of diet will significantly reduce – if not wipe out – many symptoms. Drugs and even drug-free remedies should not be looked upon as a long-term solution to faulty nutrition. We live in a society that expects doctors to write out prescriptions which overnight will put an end to all medical problems. Most of the time these drugs merely take the edge off the symptoms, suppress the problem into deeper organs and do nothing to correct the real cause. In their wake they can bring side-effects as well as deplete the body of nutrients and cause toxicity.

However, to change eating habits requires determination, a dislike of feeling ill and a positive attitude combined with patience. Rome was not built in a day and the results of years of faulty nutrition will not disappear overnight. Some people find that improvement is quick and dramatic, but for others it will take a few months for the body to adjust and benefit from the change of food. As you reduce your PMT symptoms, so you will also be greatly reducing the chances of contracting many of the other diseases which can be fatal. Moreover, if you are in charge of the food your family eats, your children will have an excellent start in life which will benefit them in later years. Husbands and boy-friends should be encouraged to join in, or at least to be supportive.

So much has been written about nutrition that in the end most of us become confused and wonder if there is anything we *can* eat! The vegetarian and vegan way of eating is gaining in popularity and has much in its favour, but as a start I propose to discuss the subject in a general way. If you wish to delve more deeply, there are plenty of books on the market, or you can make an appointment with a nutritionist. The latter is something I would recommend. Throughout this book I will be stressing that we are all individuals each of whom may have special requirements. Nutrition is a complex subject and the more research goes on, the more intricate the findings become. This chapter contains sound general advice which can be followed without concern. If you are following a diet given by your doctor, tell him/her what you are thinking of doing before changing your present regime.

You will have heard the phrase 'balance in all things' – this certainly applies to nutrition. Unfortunately the average person does not know what a balanced diet means. Really it is quite simple and by avoiding all processed foods you will be well on your way. If you eat at least half your diet raw and the rest cooked, you will be getting nearer to what is meant by a balanced diet.

The body requires forty nutrients, which have to come from the foods we eat. These are essential fatty acids, carbohydrates, complete proteins and all known minerals and vitamins. Avoiding refined foods and keeping to unprocessed natural produce ensures all these nutrients are obtained, including any which research has not yet identified.

Fats

Saturated fats are animal fats and solid at room temperature, whereas unsaturated fats (polyunsaturates) are mainly vegetable oils which remain liquid at room temperature. Much publicity has been given to eating polyunsaturated fats to lower your cholesterol levels, but unless you know you have high cholesterol levels you should consume a maximum of 25–30% of your calorie intake as fats and break your fat consumption down to 50% saturated and 50% unsaturated fats.

SATURATED FATS
These can be found in the following groups of foods – meats, dairy products (wholemilk, cream, cheeses), eggs, solid fats (butter, lard, margarines).

UNSATURATED FATS

These are made from vegetables and seeds such as corn oil, safflower oil, sunflower oil, sesame oil etc. On heating, these oils reduce their unsaturated properties and so should be used cold. Buy only cold-pressed, unhydrogenated oils and keep them in the refrigerator or they will become rancid. They are a source of Vitamin F, which cannot be made in the body but only obtained via the food we eat. Seeds, nuts and wheatgerm provide Vitamin F in its natural form, with 4–5 tablespoons of the mentioned oils per day giving optimum levels of Vitamin F.

MARGARINES

To make margarine solid the fat is hydrogenated and this manufacturing process alters the unsaturated to saturated fat. Therefore in terms of increasing your intake of polyunsaturated fats margarines are far less efficient than their advertising makes them out to be. A word of caution here about diet margarines. These are low in calories and you would probably have to eat twice as much of this type for an adequate intake of polyunsaturated fats, so diet margarine becomes an expensive buy and defeats the object of sound nutrition. It is far better to make your own Modified Butter, which tastes very good and has more essential fatty acids than margarine or butter alone. (You will find the recipe at the end of this chapter on p. 37.)

Carbohydrates

Carbohydrates are found in starches and sugar, all starches being broken down in the body to the simplest form of sugar which is then used as energy.

The conversion of starch to sugar in the intestine is sufficiently slow to give sustained energy.

Again this is an area where manufacturers have done so much damage by their refining techniques. Mainly so that the shelf life of the product is practically indefinite, flour has been refined to such an extent that there is no natural goodness left. The flour is stripped of vitamins, bran and germ and all that remains is pure starch. The only flour to buy is wholewheat, stoneground flour, but buy this in small amounts and keep in a cool place as it can go bad. Natural starch is found in grains, pulses, seeds, bulbs and tubers.

Refined sugar is also stripped of important vitamins and minerals, and unless you eat sugar cane in its raw state all types of sugar are useless from a nutritional point of view. Even commercial honey is robbed of enzymes and vitamins when heat-treated. Refined sugar causes an overproduction of insulin, upsets the alkaline digestive juices and hinders the absorption of proteins, calcium and other minerals. There is only one form of sugar that can be safely taken; this is fructose, the most common form of which is found in fruit.

Protein

A unit of protein contains twenty-two different amino acids, of which fourteen are made in the body and eight have to come from protein foods. These eight are called essential amino acids and foods which contain them are known as complete protein foods of which (in order of importance) eggs, milk, milk products, liver, meats, fish and poultry are the best sources. Other foods contain proteins, but these are not complete protein foods in that they lack some of the essential amino acids; such foods are grains, vegetables, nuts, pulses and seeds. However, combining these with eggs, milk or meat, or with each other, will give you all the essential amino acids needed.

Fruit and Vegetables

Always use fresh fruits in preference to canned, bottled or dried varieties as they supply natural sugar (fructose), potassium, carotene, Vitamin C and traces of other minerals. Avoid cooking fruit if possible as, however careful you are, the cooking process destroys nutrients. Always eat the skin of fruit if you can, as it is a good source of fibre.

Green leafy vegetables all have potassium and small amounts of vitamins and minerals. If you prefer vegetables cooked, make sure you have daily at least one of the following, lightly steamed: spinach, greens, Brussels sprouts, string beans, carrots. Vegetables are best eaten raw to avoid loss of any nutrients and from a practical point of view, there is less washing-up! On page 38 you will find the recipe for Crunchy Raw Salad including many vegetables and seeds, which really is delicious as well as being fast and easy to prepare.

Remember that fresh is preferable to frozen, but the latter can be used if you're really stuck. However, no canned vegetables please! Also bear in mind the time that elapses between the farmer dispatching his product and its arrival in the shop. You want the best and the freshest, so hand-pick everything you buy and if your grocer puts up any kind of resistance, go elsewhere. Always wash fruit and vegetables to ensure your intake of insecticides and sprays is at a minimum.

Sprouting Seeds

These seeds are valuable for their mineral, vitamin and protein content and can be grown quickly and easily in the home. Many nurseries sell them in packets with full instructions and they are ready to eat within 4–6 days. Look for fenugreek, alfalfa, mung beans and mixed sprouts, and simply add them to your salads.

Salt

An excess of salt causes water retention and hormonal imbalance as well as destroying the potassium/sodium balance. It also affects the adrenals and causes stress. As it is found naturally in the foods we eat, there is no necessity to add extra salt to food and for all PMT sufferers it should be banned from the cook-pot as well as the table. Any canned or processed foods containing salt should be promptly returned to the supermarket shelves. Kelp – an excellent source of iodine and other trace minerals – can be sprinkled on food, or potassium-based salt substitutes may also be used.

Beverages and Liquids

COFFEE AND TEA
Both these beverages contain high amounts of caffeine. Caffeine causes an increase in fatty substances in the blood and produces irritability, anxiety and mood changes – the very symptoms so commonly found in PMT sufferers. It is estimated that a cup of coffee contains 100–150 mg of caffeine, which is the equivalent of swallowing about four aspirins in caffeine content! Use decaffeinated coffee or coffee substitutes and keep to a maximum of two cups of weak tea per day.

ALCOHOL
Alcohol changes into saturated fat and is often taken as a substitute for food and to ease tension. It supplies no nutrients, only calories, and often increases the desire for sweet things. It also sends the blood sugar levels haywire and many PMT sufferers will be asleep by the second drink or feeling definitely high and light-headed.

Coffee, tea and alcohol stimulate urine production, so there is a good chance that all nutrients which dissolve in water will be lost in greater amounts through stimulation of the type brought about by these drinks.

Artificial Sweeteners

These are to be avoided, as they also trigger off the desire for sugar and are worthless nutritionally. In fact certain brands are detrimental to health.

When shopping, get used to reading the labels on food and do not buy any canned, smoked, bottled or preserved products. Anything containing refined flour, sugar, added preservatives, colourings, flavourings, salt and monosodium glutamate should be rejected. You will be surprised how little you can buy in the convenience lines! Sausages often contain sugar, as do cans of sweetcorn; many packaged meats contain preservatives – the list is endless.

To help you further, I suggest the following foods should form the basis of your shopping list:

plenty of fresh vegetables and fruit
grains and pulses
whole brown rice
wholewheat pastas
wholemeal stoneground flour
wholemeal stoneground bread
meat (in moderation), fish, poultry
eggs, low-fat cheeses, low-fat yoghurt, skimmed milk
butter or margarine of the type which can be bought in good health food stores and contains at least 15% cold-pressed oils. Better still, make your own Modified Butter (*see* p. 37) and you will have 50% cold-pressed oils!
cold-pressed unhydrogenated vegetable oils
nuts, seeds
decaffeinated coffee or coffee substitute
herb teas
unsweetened fruit juices
mineral waters.

COOKING TIPS

Never fry foods; grilling is best, but if you wish to roast meats put them on a grid so that the fat can drain off into the roasting tray. Never use the fats from meat for making gravy. When making meat, chicken or fish stocks, allow them to cool and remove all solid fat. Whenever possible, do not remove the skins from fruit and vegetables and eat them raw; when cooking, only steam-cook and serve them 'crunchy'. Never add salt to cooking. All brown rice and wholewheat pastas should be served *al dente* (slightly chewy).

If you consume the following foods you will be getting nutrients in their most concentrated form – and remember, eat at least 50% of your food *raw*.

DAILY

> 8 oz yoghurt (low-fat)
> wholegrain breads and cereals
> add wheatgerm to cereals and in cooking
> at least two whole fruits or 8 oz of pure grapefruit/orange juice
> at least 2 tablespoons of cold-pressed vegetable oils or 3 tablespoons of raw unsalted nuts
> uncooked vegetables in salads
> at least one green, leafy cooked vegetable (cabbage, spinach etc.)
> two servings of free-range poultry, fish, eggs, or low-fat cheese.

WEEKLY

> seafood, several times
> liver, once or twice
> red meat, once.

Most of us are very busy and want to ensure that we are getting the correct nutrients without having to spend hours planning menus. Here are five products to buy which can be sprinkled on food and are very beneficial to health:

> *Brewer's yeast* Contains B vitamins and is high in protein
> *Linseed* Rich in linoleic acid (an essential fatty acid)
> *Lecithin* A prime source of polyunsaturated fatty acids
> *Wheatgerm* A natural source of cholin and inosotol (B vitamins), manganese, essential fatty acids and Vitamin E
> *Kelp* A powdered form of seaweed containing many minerals, including iodine which is necessary for normal thyroid function.

Linseed, lecithin and wheatgerm can be sprinkled on all foods without altering the taste, but brewer's yeast is best put in soups or cooked dishes as it has a stronger flavour.

Eating a good balanced diet is quite simple, so here are menus to cover two days which will give you an idea of how to plan a day's eating. Recipes are given at the end of the chapter.

Breakfast
Glass of Yoghurt and Tomato Juice Cocktail
1 slice wholemeal bread with Modified Butter and a little sugarless jam (no additives or preservatives)
Decaffeinated coffee or coffee substitute with skimmed milk*

Lunch
Cold chicken with serving of Crunchy Raw Salad (see p. 38)
Wholemeal roll with Modified Butter
1 fruit
Decaffeinated coffee or coffee substitute with skimmed milk

Dinner
Vegetable Soup
Baked Fish with Parsley Sauce
At least one green leafy vegetable
Jacket potato with Modified Butter
1 fruit
Decaffeinated coffee or coffee substitute with skimmed milk

Breakfast
Glass of fresh unsweetened fruit juice
Serving of muesli (the type which has no added sugar)
Cup of decaffeinated coffee or coffee substitute with skimmed milk

Lunch
Spinach Open Omelette with mixed salad (to include lettuce, cucumber, tomatoes, watercress)
1 fruit
Cup of decaffeinated coffee or coffee substitute with skimmed milk

---

*You may, of course, substitute decaffeinated coffee with any of the following: pure fruit juice, mineral water, herb tea, or weak tea (maximum 2 cups per day).

Dinner
Fresh grapefruit
Lentil Shepherd's Pie
At least one green leafy vegetable
Serving of Healthy Dessert (see p. 41)
Cup of decaffeinated coffee or coffee substitute with skimmed milk

Daily snacks
Raw unsalted nuts, sesame seeds, pumpkin seeds, raw fruit and raw vegetables

Daily drinks
Unsweetened fruit juices, mineral waters, herb teas, a maximum of two cups of weak tea daily.

HOW TO COPE WHEN YOU'RE OUT WORKING ALL DAY
This takes a little forward planning and a couple of small food containers. First of all, make sure you get up in time to have an unrushed breakfast! I have found the easiest way to cope with lunch is to base it on a serving of Crunchy Raw Salad; this can be made the night before and put in a food box, with the cold-pressed oil and lemon juice in a separate container to be added when it's time to eat. Along with a portion of cold chicken, hard-boiled egg or low-fat cheese and a piece of fruit, this will give you a balanced meal. Unless you are very lucky, you will find your local eateries are serving mainly junk and refined foods – the same unfortunately goes for canteens. Taking along your own lunch means time saved in going out to buy food, lining up in the canteen etc., and this precious time can be spent having a leisurely walk, window-shopping, going to a lunchtime keep-fit class or whatever takes your fancy, within reason!

Keep the following in your desk drawer, briefcase or car: a large bag of raw unsalted nuts, sunflower seeds, decaffeinated coffee and herb teas. This way you won't be tempted to eat biscuits, cakes and chocolate or drink coffee and tea pumped out by machines or served well-stewed from a trolley.

SUGAR AND CARBOHYDRATE CRAVINGS

This is something many women find hard to control during the PMT phase. However, the secret in controlling the 'munchies' is to eat little and often in order to avoid a dramatic rise and fall in blood sugar levels. Also, you cut out the very foods you crave for – *sugar* and refined carbohydrates. For years I was unable to curb my appetite for chocolates, cakes, biscuits and crisps, but if you eat the way I recommend during the PMT phase you will be surprised how the cravings vanish and hunger will not be a problem. To eat little and often is the sensible way at all times, but particularly so after ovulation; eating this way does not mean weight gain – in fact, if you are overweight you will have a gradual weight loss. If you are underweight you could gain a few pounds from regular eating!

Here are some golden rules:

- 50% of your diet should be RAW
- 25–30% of your total energy should be consumed in fats (50% saturated fats and 50% unsaturated fats)
- 50% or more of your total energy intake should originate from carbohydrates
- do not consume any sugar or products containing sugar.

Your **carbo**hydrate intake should come only from the following foods:

wholemeal/wholewheat bread and bread products
wholewheat biscuits and crackers
wholegrain and fibre-rich breakfast cereals
wholemeal/wholewheat flour and flour-based products
wholewheat pasta
brown rice
vegetables and pulses
fresh and dried fruit.

The following is the type of eating pattern you should aim for, never allowing more than three hours to go by without a meal or snack.

On rising
4 oz unsweetened fruit juice

Breakfast
Serving of wholegrain or fibre-rich cereal (there are muesli-type cereals without added sugar)
1 fruit
Cup of decaffeinated coffee or coffee substitute with skimmed milk

2 hours after breakfast
4 oz skimmed milk

1 hour before lunch
Snack of raw, unsalted nuts and/or seeds

Lunch
1 slice wholemeal bread with Modified Butter
Mixed raw salad, or selection of vegetables with cold chicken
1 fruit
Cup of decaffeinated coffee or coffee substitute with skimmed milk

3 hours after lunch
4 oz skimmed milk

1 hour before dinner
4 oz unsweetened fruit juice

Dinner
Vegetable Soup
Spaghetti with Tuna Fish Sauce
1 fruit
Decaffeinated coffee or coffee substitute with skimmed milk

2–3 hours after dinner
Snack of raw unsalted nuts mixed with a few raisins

Bedtime
Wholemeal roll with Modified Butter, filled with salad and low fat cheese

Not permitted
Alcohol, sugar in any form (pastries, biscuits etc.), coffee, salt, more than two cups of weak tea (substitute herb teas and mineral waters).

Nutrition is a very complex subject and there is a wide variety of books available, written for easy reading. It is important to remember that each one of us is unique and this chapter is handling the subject in general terms. I would strongly recommend that if you are still feeling under par after following my advice for two to three months, you should go a step further and make an appointment with a holistic centre where your individual needs can be diagnosed and corrected.

This approach to eating will be a new way of life and you may be wondering how to cope with the shopping and cooking. Get organized, make out a list of necessities from the list given in this chapter, then with the aid of a good health cookbook, pick out the recipes that appeal to you, add these ingredients to your list and off you go! There are many delicious meals which can be prepared quickly and easily. As you become more attuned to your body, you will quickly learn that eating the wrong foods only aggravates your symptoms and this will provide enough inspiration to keep you going! If you take a quick look at Chapter 11, you will find case histories which include women who were suffering severe symptoms of PMT, yet a change of diet got rid of the symptoms in the first month! No drugs or remedies were involved.

Finally, the following is an extreme example of a woman suffering from PMT, but it is important to note that nutrition was mentioned in court:

In a recent court case, a woman was conditionally discharged after admitting killing her lover by running him down in a car. She pleaded guilty of manslaughter on the grounds of diminished responsibility due to PMT. Her doctor said in court that it was a vital factor that she had not eaten for nine hours and the syndrome had caused an accumulation of adrenalin in the blood which led to irritability, aggression, impatience and loss of self-control. The doctor was quoted in the newspaper report of the case as saying it was this which was the primary cause of his patient's actions.

Recipes

Modified Butter

225 g/8 oz butter
1/2 cup safflower oil (cold-pressed/unrefined)

Put the butter out to soften at room temperature. Place in a liquidizer and add the safflower oil; blend well, place in a suitable container and keep in the fridge.

Salad Dressing

1 clove garlic
3 dessertspoons safflower oil (cold-pressed/unrefined)
1 dessertspoon fresh lemon juice
little sea salt (optional)
pinch of mixed herbs

Cut the clove of garlic in half and rub around the salad bowl. Add all the other ingredients and mix well.

Vegetable Soup   Serves 4

This soup avoids using fat and overcooking the vegetables.

1.1 l/2 pints chicken stock with all fat removed
25 g/1 oz cooked brown rice
4 carrots, diced
1 cauliflower broken into small florets
pinch of sea salt (optional)
parsley

Steam-cook the vegetables until just tender. Heat the stock and add the brown rice. Add the vegetables and sea-salt but do not boil. Garnish with chopped parsley.

Yoghurt and Tomato Juice Cocktail   Serves 1

1 small carton low-fat yoghurt
empty yoghurt carton of tomato juice
juice of half a lemon
1/2–1 teaspoon brewer's yeast

Put all the ingredients in a blender and mix thoroughly. This is an appetizing way of taking brewer's yeast and gives complete protein.

Crunchy Raw Salad

Serving: Use quantities according to the number you are serving.

Lettuce, radishes, green pepper,
tomatoes, cucumber, mushrooms,
cauliflower, carrots, pumpkin and
sunflower seeds, raw unsalted nuts. For
each serving add 1 teaspoon each of
wheatgerm, lecithin and linseed

Thoroughly wash all vegetables. Scrub the carrots – do not peel. Chop into bite-size pieces and place in a bowl. Add the wheatgerm, lecithin and linseed. Mix with the Salad Dressing on p. 37. Stir well and serve immediately. You can of course use any raw vegetables for this salad, also any sprouting seeds if you have grown them. You can make this salad in large quantities, omitting the Salad Dressing, and keep it in the refrigerator covered in cling-film; it will stay fresh for up to two days.

Parsley Sauce

15 g/½ oz Modified Butter
15 g/½ oz wholemeal flour
300 ml/½ pint cold skimmed
   milk
sea salt (optional)

pepper
3–4 tablespoons chopped
   fresh parsley
pinch of ground nutmeg

Melt the Modified Butter in a heavy-based saucepan until foamy. Stir in the flour and cook slowly for 3 minutes, stirring all the time. Remove from heat and add the milk, stirring until smooth. Return to the heat and cook until the sauce thickens, stirring all the time. Simmer over a low heat for 3 more minutes, add seasonings and parsley. Stir well and serve with baked fish.

Baked Fish

Serves 2

2 large plaice
100 g/4 oz mushrooms, finely chopped
15 g/1 oz Modified Butter
1 small onion, finely chopped
sea salt (optional)
ground black pepper

Melt the Modified Butter in a pan and cook the chopped onion until golden. Add the mushrooms and cook for 15–20 minutes. Add the seasoning, stir well and remove from heat. Cut the plaice in half lengthwise and spread the mushroom and onion mixture on the skinned side of the fish. Roll up the fish and place them in a baking dish with ¼ pint water. Put a piece of greaseproof paper or tinfoil on top and bake in the oven (180°C/350°F/Gas Mark 4) for approximately 20 minutes. Serve with parsley sauce.

Spinach Open Omelette   Serves 1

2 eggs
1 small onion, finely chopped
6 large raw spinach leaves (remove stalks and chop finely)
1 dessertspoon Modified Butter
freshly-milled black pepper

Melt the butter in a frying pan and cook onions until soft. Heat the grill to its highest setting. Place the chopped spinach on top of the onions. Beat the eggs with a fork and add the freshly-milled black pepper. Turn the heat on full under the frying pan and add the eggs. Using a fork or palette knife draw the outside of the omelette inwards, allowing the liquid egg to run to the edges of the pan. Place the pan under the grill to set the top. Serve with mixed salad.

Spaghetti with Tuna Fish Sauce   Serves 4

2 tablespoons Modified Butter
1 clove garlic, chopped
1 × 200-g/7-oz tin tuna fish in brine
3 tablespoons chopped fresh parsley
2 tablespoons tomato purée

230 ml/8 fluid oz fish stock
sea salt (optional)
freshly ground black pepper
1/2 kg/1 lb wholewheat spaghetti

Heat the Modified Butter in a saucepan and add the garlic. Cook for one minute. Drain the tuna fish and break up into small pieces. Add to the garlic along with parsley, tomato purée and stock. Season. Cook the wholewheat spaghetti in boiling water until *al dente*. Drain and mix with tuna sauce. Garnish with chopped parsley.

Lentil Shepherd's Pie

Serves 4–6

170 g/6 oz brown lentils
600 ml/1 pint water
1 bayleaf
1 onion, finely chopped
1 garlic clove, crushed
1 small carrot, finely chopped
100 g/4 oz mushrooms, finely
  chopped
1 tablespoon safflower oil
  (cold-pressed)

400 g/14 oz fresh tomatoes,
  skinned and chopped
sea salt (optional)
freshly ground black pepper
1/2–1 kg/1–2 lb mashed potato
  (using Modified Butter and
  skimmed milk)
15 g/1 oz grated cheese
  (low-fat)

Place the lentils and bayleaf in a saucepan with the water and simmer for 45–60 minutes. Heat the oven to 200°C/400°F/Gas Mark 6. Cook the onion in the oil for 10 minutes and add carrot, mushrooms and garlic; cook for a further 3 minutes, stirring all the time. Remove from heat and add tomatoes and seasoning. Place the mixture in a well-greased ovenproof dish and cover with mashed potatoes. Sprinkle with grated cheese and bake for 50 minutes. Serve with spinach or Brussels sprouts.

Healthy Dessert

Serves 4

1 large tub low-fat yoghurt
1 tablespoon tahini (ground sesame seeds)
1 dessertspoon linseed and lecithin
12 almonds
1 sliced banana
1 chopped apple

Place all the ingredients in a liquidizer and blend thoroughly. Serve this dessert immediately.

CHAPTER FIVE

Weight Loss can be Easy – When you Know How!

Does any of this sound like you?

- Whenever I go on a diet, I feel ill and hungry.
- Diets are fine for the first two/three weeks of my cycle.
- On the run-up to my period, all my good intentions are ruined. I just have to eat chocolates/biscuits – whatever I can lay my hands on.
- I've a wardrobe full of clothes that don't fit.
- I won't buy new clothes until I've lost weight.
- I often go around with the top button of my jeans/skirts etc. undone.
- I've lost interest in my appearance.
- I hate myself fat.
- I've no energy – especially for exercise.

If you can relate to any of these remarks, then something must be done! We need to like ourselves before we can enjoy the world around us; just as important are all the health reasons for not carting around excess pounds. The death rate rises dramatically with increased weight, and although weight itself may not be the primary cause of many diseases it certainly worsens the situation. In general people who live to a ripe old age tend to be sensible with their diet, physically active and underweight rather than over-weight.

Many women who do not consider themselves overweight will experience an increase in weight prior to their period. This can be anything from a few pounds to a stone! It is due to water retention and the weight normalizes at the onset of menstruation. Avoiding salt and refined foods can very effectively reduce this problem in many cases. However, difficulties occur when there is an over-whelming desire for fattening foods which over a period of time has caused an overall weight gain. Dieting then becomes a real hassle. The period begins, a new diet is started and the weight begins to drop off. Then just as you are doing well – it's premen-strual tension time and the pounds are back yet again. This is a very depressing experience to go through month after month and many women give up the 'battle of the bulge'.

So here is some good news for anyone with a weight problem.

- You can drop pounds steadily *throughout* the month.
- You won't need to alter your basic diet (provided, of course, you are following the general advice in Chapter 4).
- You won't feel hungry.

Sounds almost too good to be true? The secret is *soluble fibre*. Before you think you already know all about fibre, let me explain about exciting news which has come out of recent research.

There are different types of fibre and one which has been mentioned frequently over the past few years is wheatbran. Did you know that high levels of bran can cause intestinal irritation, constipation, anaemia and the loss of important minerals from your tissues? Wheatbran and wholegrains contain mainly insolu-ble fibre and remain as separate particles despite liquid being added.

Soluble fibre swells when liquid is added and is fermentable – in other words the bacteria in the intestines can digest it. This gives a sense of fullness and satisfaction. Research has shown that soluble fibre seems to aid the absorption of water-soluble vitamins as well as stabilizing blood sugar levels by transporting sugars further down into the bowel and slowing down the rate of absorption. As the soluble fibre itself is not digested, it does not matter how much of this type of fibre is consumed – your calorie intake is not increased!

Soluble fibres can help to prevent diabetes and cardio-vascular disease and also lower blood cholesterol. They will also aid slimmers by stopping the hunger pangs which so often cause diets to be broken.

In the UK we consume on average 20 g of fibre per day, making us one of the lowest fibre consumers in the world. In Africa and Asia the consumption of fibre is approximately 40–60 g daily. In these societies the major killer diseases are virtually unknown – so is obesity! On the basis of available evidence, it seems that carbohydrate intake need not be kept low, if the majority of carbohydrate is complex and high fibre foods are consumed.

All carbohydrates, sugars and starches are converted into blood sugar, refined carbohydrates being more quickly converted. A change to a diet high in soluble fibres will:

1 slow down the rate of absorption of end products produced by carbohydrates
2 actually inhibit the digestion of carbohydrates.

The Sources of Soluble Fibre

Pectin is a good source of soluble fibre, and is found in fresh fruits – particularly in apples. It has been found to increase fat in the stools, and naturally helps to eliminate toxic waste material from the body. Pectin also helps to develop bacterial flora which are required for the proper assimilation of nutrients from food. Other good sources of soluble fibre are vegetables, seeds, nuts, legumes such as oatmeal, kidney beans, etc.

You can slim simply by increasing these foods in your eating plan. An addition of 6 g soluble fibre per day should be enough to reduce your weight without making other drastic changes.

To help you select foods high in fibre, here is a list of foods which are valuable in a healthy weight-loss eating plan. Remember to eat them raw whenever possible.

SOURCES OF FIBRE	FIBRE CONTENT PER 100 g	SOURCES OF FIBRE	FIBRE CONTENT PER 100 g
Almonds	14.3	Loganberries	6.2
Apples	2.0	Low-fat soya	
Baked potatoes	2.5	flour	14.3

SOURCES OF FIBRE	FIBRE CONTENT PER 100 g	SOURCES OF FIBRE	FIBRE CONTENT PER 100 g
Beansprouts	3.0	Mung beans	6.4
Beetroot	2.5	Mushrooms	2.5
Blackberries	7.3	Oatmeal (raw)	7.0
Blackcurrants	8.7	Oranges	2.0
Brazil nuts	9.0	Parsley leaves	9.1
Broad beans	4.2	Parsnips	2.5
Broccoli	4.1	Passion fruit	15.9
Brussels sprouts	2.9	Peanuts	8.1
Butter beans	5.1	Pearl barley	2.2
Carrots	3.1	Prunes (raw)	16.1
Cauliflower	2.1	Raisins	6.8
Celeriac	4.9	Red cabbage (raw)	3.4
Chick peas	5.2	Red kidney beans	25.0
Dried apricots	24.0	Runner beans	3.4
Dried dates	8.7	Spinach	6.3
Dried figs	18.5	Spring greens	3.8
Dried peaches	14.3	Sultanas	7.0
Dried peas	4.8	Sweetcorn	4.7
Fresh apricots	2.1	Turnips	2.2
Fresh peas	5.2	Watercress	3.3
Haricot beans	7.4	White cabbage (raw)	3.4
Hazelnuts	6.1	Wholemeal bread	9.6
Horseradish (raw)	8.3	Wholemeal flour	9.6
Lemons (whole)	5.2		
Lentils	3.7		

(*Source: The Composition of Foods* by A. A. Paul and D. A. T. Southgate (McCance & Widdowson))

If you are not prepared to increase your fibre consumption with the foods suggested, you can increase your soluble fibre with Lejguar, a brand name of *guar gum* which comes from the Indian cluster bean. Guar gum has been used for many years by food manufacturers as a thickener and emulsion stabilizer. In 1974, medical researchers became interested in the product when dietary fibre was found to be of benefit to health and disease. The fact that certain types of dietary fibre were observed to have considerable effects on glucose and insulin responses to meals led to the product of Lejguar.

Dr Marcin Krotkiewski ran a clinical trial at Sahlgren's Hospital in Sweden, using guar gum for the management of obese patients. *These patients were told not to alter their eating patterns*. During a ten-week period the patients reported reduced hunger, and weight losses of up to fourteen pounds.

Lejguar comes in 250-g packs, in granular form, containing approximately 90% guar gum. It is natural and harmless and the granules have a neutral taste. This product is available from chemists, and if your doctor considers you must reduce your weight for health reasons, it can be prescribed on the National Health.

You should never consider Lejguar as an alternative to a good diet, but as an addition. A balanced approach to nutrition should be your first priority. The addition of soluble fibre in your diet, plus a three-hourly eating plan, avoiding sugar and refined carbohydrates, will help to curb those food cravings; then weight loss need not be an impossible achievement.

CHAPTER SIX

Vitamins, Minerals and Dietary Supplements

There are a number of vitamins which are important in the management of PMT and if you follow the advice given in the nutritional chapter and eat a well-balanced diet you will be getting most of your requirements. However, as it can be difficult to find really fresh food, there is always a possibility that certain deficiencies may occur. Again this is an area of confusion, with many doctors stating that there is no need to take extra vitamins and that these can be dangerous. The latter is true for certain vitamins, and it is good practice never to take megadoses of supplements without discussing your requirements with a qualified naturopath. If you are taking a number at one time, and are in any doubt, stop for a couple of days; then recommence and take them one by one to see which vitamin is causing the problem. Most women, provided they do not exceed the recommended dosages, should find everything plain sailing.

Vitamins are prepared as tablets, capsules, powders and liquids:

Tablets These are the most convenient form, as the shelf-life is longer and they are easier to store and carry.

Capsules Again easy to store and are used for oil-soluble vitamins such as A, D and E.

Powders These have extra potency and are devoid of additives, binders and fillers.

Liquids Liquids are best for those who find tablets and capsules difficult to swallow. They can be mixed easily with drinks.

If you are watching your fat intake or find you break out in spots prior to your period, you are perhaps wise to avoid capsules and take your vitamins in dry form.

Both synthetic and natural vitamins work very well. However Dr Therou G. Randolph, who works with allergies, has said, 'A synthetically derived substance may cause a reaction in a chemically susceptible person when the same material of natural origin is tolerated, despite the two substances having identical chemical structures.'

If we take Vitamin C, in its synthetic form it is ascorbic acid only, whereas natural Vitamin C contains bioflavonoids, making the Vitamin C much more effective.

Chelated minerals Since many people do not digest their food correctly, it is always sensible to buy minerals in this form, as they have been specially manufactured for easy digestion.

Time release Vitamins are manufactured in a way that releases them over a period of time. As most vitamins are water soluble they cannot be stored in the body, but by taking time-release vitamins there is minimal loss and over a 24-hour period blood levels remain stable.

Kept under cool, dark conditions, unopened vitamins have a shelf life of about three years. Opened, but in the same conditions, vitamins will remain unspoilt for a year.

Vitamins and minerals should be taken together for proper absorption, and it is best to split your supplements throughout the day. Always take them after food, as water soluble vitamins such as B and C can leave the body two hours later if taken on an empty stomach.

As it is always better to take vitamins and minerals in their natural form, I have included a list of foods which are the best sources for each individual supplement.

There are a number of vitamins and minerals which are important for the management of PMT. Please be sure that you are eating a balanced selection of the foods mentioned by each supplement, and also following the nutritional advice given in the previous chapter. If you still have stubborn symptoms, you can increase your consumption of suitable foods and take vitamin supplements that will help.

B Vitamins

It is best to take B vitamins together, so look carefully at the labels and make sure you are buying a product which gives you adequate amounts of each B vitamin. The following are the vitamins contained in a B complex:

Thiamine (B1)
Riboflavin (B2)
Niacin (B3)
Biotin
Pantothenic acid (B5)
Pyridoxine (B6)
Para-aminobenzoic acid
Choline
Inositol
Cyanacobalamin (B12)
Folic acid

If your chosen B complex contains 100 mg of B1 and 100 mg of B6, you can be sure that the rest of the vitamins are balanced.

Emotional stress can cause a loss of B vitamins, resulting in irritability and fatigue. Choline and inositol assist the liver in breaking down fatty foods and fat-soluble hormones such as oestrogen. Inositol has a tranquillizing effect on the central nervous system, which may help with irritability and anxiety. Choline and inositol are found in:

Brewer's yeast, wheatgerm, liver, wholegrains, milk, citrus fruits, lecithin, egg yolks, soya beans.

Finally, I have given more details on three of the B vitamins, B1, B2 and B6, as this particular combination (with the doses mentioned) has worked well for many women, particularly if they have also followed the nutritional advice.

Vitamins For PMT

ARDDA = Adult Recommended Daily Dietary Allowance
PMT = Suggested Daily Allowance for PMT

VITAMIN	ARDDA/ PMT	GOOD FOR	NATURAL SOURCES	NEED MORE/NEED LESS
A In its complete form is known as retinol and is found in animal, fish and dairy products; in plants occurs in the form of carotene	ARDDA 2500 IU (can be toxic in large doses – over 100,000 IU daily)	Acne, oily skin and hair	Carrots, spinach, watercress, cabbage, green salads, butter, egg yolk, liver, fish-liver oils, milk, nuts, tomatoes, apricots, melons, rose-hips, oranges	Less if you are eating a balanced diet containing plenty of the listed foods; are on the contraceptive pill; more if you are using a zinc supplement; are not augmenting polyunsaturated fats by vitamins C and E
B1 (Thiamin) Water soluble – excess amounts	ARDDA 1 mg; PMT 100 mg	Nervous system, mental attitude; the digestion,	Brewer's yeast, rice husks (whole brown	More if you smoke; are a moderate to heavy drinker; are

are excreted by the body; destroyed by the heat of cooking		especially carbohydrates; water retention – has a mildly diuretic action	rice), bran, wheatgerm, oatmeal, nuts, seeds, milk, meat, liver, poultry, most vegetables	taking the contraceptive pill; live mainly on low calorie foods such as cottage cheese, fruit juice and salads; drink plenty of coffee; eat significant amounts of processed and refined foods and sugar; take sulphur drugs
B2 (Riboflavin) Water soluble – excess amounts are excreted by the body; not destroyed by the cooking process	ARDDA 1.3 mg; PMT 10 mg twice a day	Utilization of carbohydrates, fats and proteins	Milk, liver, kidney, brewer's yeast, brown rice, eggs, fish, leafy green vegetables and kelp	*More* if you are under stress and strain; rarely eat meat and dairy products; are taking the contraceptive pill; are a moderate to heavy drinker; take sulphur drugs

VITAMIN	ARDDA/ PMT	GOOD FOR	NATURAL SOURCES	NEED MORE/NEED LESS
B6 (Pyridoxine) Water soluble – excess amounts are excreted by the body; only remains in the body for eight hours after ingestion	ARDDA 2 mg; PMT 100 mg	The assimilation of protein and fat; aiding the conversion of tryptophan to niacin; helping prevent nervous disorders; regulation of fluid retention, mood swings, irritability, breast tenderness, fatigue and sugar craving	Brewer's yeast, wheatgerm, bran, Blackstrap molasses, liver, kidney, heart, cabbage, egg yolks, nuts, tomatoes, bananas, avocado pears	*More* if you are on the contraceptive pill; eat large amounts of protein; eat a diet high in processed foods; overcook food; are a moderate to heavy drinker
C Water soluble; as the body cannot make	ARDDA 60 mg; PMT 600 mg	Water retention – has a diuretic action; protecting	Citrus fruits (fresh), rose-hips, blackcurrants,	*More* if you are taking any drugs or antibiotics; live in an urban area with

| vitamin C it has to come from food; leaves the body within two to three hours | against harmful chemicals and pollutants; assisting in the formation of collagen; promoting the body's absorption of iron; anti-stress | strawberries, tomatoes, cauliflower, potatoes, green peppers and green leafy vegetables | carbon monoxide fumes and lead pollution; are a heavy smoker; take the contraceptive pill |

VITAMIN	ARDDA/ PMT	GOOD FOR	NATURAL SOURCES	NEED MORE/NEED LESS
E Fat soluble and stored in fatty tissue, although storage is of short duration; *warning*: should be taken at least eight hours before or after supplements containing inorganic iron (ferrous sulphate) as inorganic iron destroys Vitamin E	ARDDA not established; PMT 200 IU daily	Acting as an anti-oxidant for polyunsaturated fatty acids; protecting other nutrients such as Vitamin A from oxidation; alleviating fatigue; water retention – has a diuretic action; retarding cellular ageing due to oxidation	Whole, raw sprouted seeds and nuts, wheatgerm, soya beans, cold-pressed vegetable oils, broccoli, spinach, Brussels sprouts, leafy green vegetables, wholegrain cereals, eggs	*More* if you are on a diet high in polyunsaturated oils; have chlorinated drinking water; are taking hormones or the contraceptive pill; are taking high doses of Vitamin C

Minerals for PMT

MINERAL	ARDDA/PMT	GOOD FOR	NATURAL SOURCES	NEED MORE/NEED LESS
CALCIUM	ARDDA 800 mg; PMT 800 mg	Maintaining strong bones and normal muscle tone; helping prevent period cramps and pain	Milk and milk products, soya beans, sardines, salmon, peanuts, walnuts, sunflower seeds, dried beans, green vegetables	*More* if you consume large quantities of fat; oxalic acid (found in rhubarb and chocolate); phyticacid (found in grains)

MINERAL	ARDDA/PMT	GOOD FOR	NATURAL SOURCES	NEED MORE/NEED LESS
MAGNESIUM *Note:* Dolomite is a natural form of calcium and magnesium which does not require Vitamin D for assimilation; 5 dolomite tablets are the equivalent of 750 mg of calcium	ARDDA 300–400 mg; PMT 350 mg	Fighting depression; increasing calcium absorption; normalizing glucose metabolism; decreasing menstrual cramps	Nuts, almonds, seeds, dark green vegetables, apples, figs, lemon, grapefruit, soya beans, wholewheat flour, chicken, lentils	*More* if you are a moderate to heavy drinker; are on the contraceptive pill; *less* magnesium if you eat plenty of nuts; live in an area with hard water
POTASSIUM	ARDDA not established; PMT 600 mg	Regulating the body's water balance; normalizing heart rhythms; potassium loss	Citrus fruits (fresh), watercress, green leafy vegetables, sunflower seeds,	*More* if you are under mental and physical stress; are taking diuretic drugs; are a moderate to heavy consumer of alcohol,

				coffee, sugar
		due to hypoglycaemia	bananas, potatoes	
ZINC Note: if you add zinc to your diet, you will need more Vitamin A	ARDDA 15 mg; PMT up to 25 mg	The maintenance of enzyme systems and cells; controlling an overabundance of copper, which can increase levels of oestrogen and cause moodiness; helping mental alertness	Wheatgerm, brewer's yeast, pumpkin seeds, eggs, ground mustard, non-fat dried milk, chicken, brown rice, lentils, wholewheat flour, soya meal	More if you take large amounts of Vitamin B6; are a heavy drinker; have irregular periods
EVENING PRIMROSE OIL The richest natural source of gamma-linolenic	PMT mild to moderate symptoms: Efamol PMP pack taken 10 days before	Regulating the menstrual cycle; promoting healthy skin; maintaining normal	Safflower seed oil, sunflower seed oil, corn oil, nuts, seeds, wheatgerm	More if you eat a westernized diet of refined foods; eat a diet rich in saturated fats; have a moderate to high intake of

MINERAL	ARDDA/ PMT	GOOD FOR	NATURAL SOURCES	NEED MORE/NEED LESS
acid (GLA) (refer to Chapter 1 for clinical trial result)	period begins; pack includes: Evening Primrose oil plus vitamin supplement; *moderate to severe symptoms*: 2 × 500 mg capsules 3 times a day after food for 2–3 months (can be reduced as symptoms improve); to be taken in conjunction with Efavite – a mineral and vitamin supplement	cholesterol levels; helping the free flow of blood; regulating blood pressure		alcohol; are diabetic; lack zinc, magnesium and Vitamin B6

CHAPTER SEVEN

Homoeopathy and Homoeopathic Remedies

For many years homoeopathic medicines have been used as a safe and effective means of treating both serious and minor ailments. Homoeopathy is derived from the Greek word *homoios*, meaning 'like'. The principle of this type of treatment is that 'like cures like'. In other words, the illness is treated with a substance that produces the same symptoms as those displayed by the person who is ill. The remedies seek to stimulate and not suppress the body's reaction against illness. Treating the patient and not the illness assists the patient to regain health by stimulating the body's natural forces of recovery.

People vary in their response to an illness according to their basic temperament, and this is one of the principles of homoeopathy. Therefore patients suffering from the same diseases often require different remedies. On the other hand, a group of patients with different diseases may all benefit from the same remedy.

The principle of homoeopathy was known to Hippocrates, the fifth-century B.C. Greek physician, and to the Swiss alchemist Paracelsus in the sixteenth century, both of whom recognized the role of nature as the curer of diseases. During the sixteenth and seventeenth centuries the principle 'let like be treated by like' was often mentioned by physicians, but homoeopathy as it is practised today owes its establishment to Dr Samuel Hahnemann, a German physician, scholar and chemist who lived during the late eighteenth and early nineteenth century. Believing that existing medical practices often did more harm than good, he sought to find a method that would be safe, gentle and effective. As human beings have a capacity to heal themselves, the symptoms of disease reflecting the individual's struggle to overcome illness, he sought to discover and if possible remove the cause of the trouble by stimulating the body's natural healing power.

Dr Hahnemann worked with remedies obtained from animal, vegetable and mineral sources. More rarely, biological materials were effective in extreme dilutions; this was very noticeable in the case of poisons, which could produce symptoms similar to those of certain illnesses. In very diluted doses they suggested themselves as remedies on the 'like cures like' principle. Over a considerable period of time Hahnemann and his followers took small doses of various poisonous substances and noted the symptoms produced. These were called 'provings'. They then treated patients suffering from similar symptoms with these substances; the results were encouraging and at times remarkable.

To avoid side effects, Hahnemann worked to establish the smallest effective dose and in doing so found that the more diluted a remedy, the more effective it became. From this arose the three principles of homoeopathy:

1 A medicine which in large doses produces symptoms of a disease, will in small doses cure that disease.
2 By extreme dilution, the medicine's curative properties are enhanced and all poisonous or undesirable side effects are lost.
3 Homoeopathic medicines are prescribed individually by the study of the whole person, according to temperament and responses.

Today homoeopathy has been developed in many countries of the world to the point where it is formally accepted as a safe and effective form of alternative medical treatment. In Britain it is used by some members of the Royal Family and is recognized by Act of Parliament, all homoeopathic medicines being available on prescription under the National Health Service; as medicines they are widely recognized as a safe and effective alternative to the conventional types. Prepared to impeccable modern standards of quality from pure natural sources, they are pleasant and sweet-tasting. As the remedies are completely safe they can be given to children and even babies, so should you decide you wish to try any of the suggested preparations you can do so without concern. However, it is important to emphasize that if any symptoms persist beyond a reasonable period of time and you wish to continue with homoeopathic treatment, then expert advice should be sought from a homoeopathic doctor.

It is possible to purchase a wide range of homoeopathic medicines from chemists, health food stores or direct from the manufacturers.

The most common homoeopathic medicines are:

1	*Aconitum napellus*	(Aconite)
2	*Actaea racemosa*	(Actaea rac.)
3	*Apis mellifioa*	(Apis mel.)
4	*Argentum nitricum*	(Argent. nit.)
5	*Arnica montana*	(Arnica)
6	*Arsenicum album*	(Arsen. Alb.)
7	*Belladonna*	(Belladonna)
8	*Bryonia alba*	(Bryonia)
9	*Calcarea carbonica*	(Calc. carb.)
10	*Calcarea fluorica*	(Calc. fluor.)
11	*Calcarea phosphorica*	(Calc. phos.)
12	*Cantharis vesicatoria*	(Cantharis)
13	*Carbo vegetabilis*	(Carbo veg.)
14	*Cuprum metallicum*	(Cuprum met.)
15	*Drosera rotundifolia*	(Drosera)
16	*Euphrasia officinalis*	(Euphrasia)
17	*Ferrum phosphoricum*	(Ferr. phos.)
18	*Gelsemium sempervirens*	(Gelsemium)
19	*Graphites*	(Graphites)
20	*Hamamelis virginica*	(Hamamelis)
21	*Hepar sulphuris*	(Hepar sulph.)
22	*Hypericum perforatum*	(Hypericum)
23	*Ignatia amara*	(Ignatia)
24	*Ipecacuanha*	(Ipecac.)
25	*Kalium bichromicum*	(Kali. bich.)
26	*Kalium phosphoricum*	(Kali. phos.)
27	*Lycopodium clavatum*	(Lycopodium)
28	*Mercurius solubilis*	(Merc. sol.)
29	*Natrum muriaticum*	(Nat. mur.)

30	*Nux vomica*	(Nux vom.)
31	Phosphorus	(Phosphorus)
32	*Pulsatilla nigricans*	(Pulsatilla)
33	*Rhus toxicodendron*	(Rhus tox.)
34	*Ruta graveolens*	(Ruta grav.)
35	Sepia	(Sepia)
36	*Silicea*	(Silicea)
37	Sulphur	(Sulphur)
38	*Thuja occidentalis*	(Thuja)

Homoeopathic medicines come in various potencies, but for home use the sixth potency is normally used, and this is shown on the bottle with a figure 6 after the name of the medicine (e.g. Pulsatilla 6).

The frequency of dose should be:

Acute conditions 2 tablets every 2 hours for six doses, then 2 tablets 3 times per day between meals for three days.
Chronic cases 2 tablets 3 times per day until relief is obtained.

If symptoms appear on a regular basis, the chosen remedy can be taken one week before the monthly period and continued three or four days into the period. This may be repeated every month until improvement is experienced.

Watch your response to each dose, and when improvement is evident increase the interval between doses, continue for two more days and then *Stop*. Repeat only if the original symptoms recur. Always stop when the condition has cleared.

If after taking a remedy there is a worsening of the symptoms, *Stop* and do not repeat the medication. Only repeat if the original symptoms recur.

Homoeopathic medicines are best taken apart from food and drink. They should be dissolved on a clean tongue, free from the effects of tobacco or strongly flavoured toothpastes. Always keep your remedies in a cool place and away from strong-smelling items.

You will find those medicines which help you by experience. There may be one particular remedy which will always bring relief, regardless of the symptoms you are experiencing.

Self-treatment with homoeopathic medicines is relatively straightforward. The following guide is in two parts. The first section is an alphabetical Index of Symptoms relating to PMT. When you have looked up a specific symptom, then refer to the second section, the List of Medicines. By cross reference between the two lists, you can then select the appropriate medicine which most closely matches your total symptoms picture and (where mentioned) appearance and temperament.

Index Of Symptoms

SYMPTOMS		MEDICATION
ANXIETY	Sudden panic attacks	Aconite
	More prolonged, with periodic panic attacks	Arsen. alb.
	With fainting spells	Sulphur
	With profuse sweating	Sulphur
APPETITE EXCESSIVE	Feeling of emptiness even after a meal	Calc. carb.
	Varies greatly to complete loss of appetite	Ferr. phos.
	Even at night, but is easily satisfied	Lycopodium
BREAST TENDERNESS		Calc. carb.
CONFUSION	Associated with depression and despondency	Actaea rac.
DEPRESSION	Associated with confusion and despondency	Actaea rac.
	In emotional individuals and because of bereavement	Ignatia
	Especially women who are easily depressed	Sepia

SYMPTOMS		MEDICATION
FAT EXCESS	With excessive appetite	Calc. carb.
	Often accompanied by unhealthy skin	Graphites
	In shy and emotional individuals	Pulsatilla
FLUID RETENTION	Heaviness of breasts with symptoms relieved by flow; usually accompanied by inability to tolerate tight clothes and are worse in the morning	Lachesis (This remedy is not one of the commonly found homoeopathic preparations but can be ordered by post, *see* Chapter 12)
HEADACHES	With painful watering eyes and unable to bear bright light	Euphrasia
	With humming in the ears	Kali. phos.
	Hammering headache preceded by misty vision or zig-zag lights (*see* Migraine)	Nat. mur.
IRRITABILITY	From jealousy, fright, anger or grief	Apis mel.
	With impulsiveness	Argent. nit.
	Very ill-tempered and easily aggravated	Bryonia
	Extreme irritability	Nux vom.

SYMPTOMS		MEDICATION
MIGRAINE	Preceded by misty vision or zig-zag lights	Nat. mur.
	Beginning in the neck coming over the head and ending in one eye	Silicea
		Ignatia
	Blurred vision before headache	Kali. bich.
	(A homoeopathic medicine 'Feverfew' has been available in the last year. Used by migraine sufferers, it has had very good results.)	
SUGAR/ CARBO- HYDRATE CRAVINGS	With feelings of irritability, melancholia and excessive hunger	Lycopodium

List Of Homoeopathic Medicines

As each homoeopathic remedy has a number of uses, all PMT symptoms are in italic type to make identification easier. Other symptoms (not PMT-related) are listed; if you purchase a remedy for PMT, it is a pity not to know the other uses to which it can be put.

Remember to choose the preparation which overall matches your total symptoms picture and (where mentioned) appearance and temperament.

MEDICINE	AILMENT/CONDITION	SYMPTOMS WORSEN/IMPROVE	NOTES
ACONITE (Aconitum napellus)	Anxiety Will also help: symptoms which are sudden, violent and brief; exposure to draughts or a cold wind; dry, suffocating cough; asthma; sore throat following exposure to cold winds; high temperature with great thirst; great pain; bereavement; animal bites; restlessness, fear, grief	Worsen at midnight; when lying on affected side; in a warm room; in tobacco smoke; in cold winds; when listening to music; improve in the open air; with bedclothes thrown off	
ACTAEA RAC. (Actaea racemosa)	Confusion, Depression Will also help: headache; stiff neck; neuralgia; painful muscles following strenuous exercise; shooting pains	Worsen in cold and damp; when moving; improve in warmth; when eating; headache improves in open air	Helpful for depression, confusion and despondency caused by over-exertion or fright

	Irritability	Worsen/Improve	Additional notes
APIS MEL. (*Apis mellifica*)	*Irritability* (from jealousy, fright, anger or grief) Will also help: burning stinging pains; swelling of lower eyelids; absence of thirst; effects of insect stings	*Worsen* (symptoms mostly on the right side) during late afternoon; after sleeping; from heat; when touched; in airless and heated rooms; *improve* in open air; from cold bathing	
ARGENT. NIT. (*Argentum nitricum*)	*Irritability* Will also help: acidity, dyspepsia; headache; conjunctivitis; craving for sweet food, cheese, fats or salt, followed by upset stomach with much flatulence; dizziness from overwork and mental strain	*Worsen* in warmth; after eating sweet foods; from overwork; with worry about the future	Suited to impulsive, irritable or nervous people who tend to worry about the uncertainties of the future. Helpful when taken before a difficult undertaking (e.g. making a speech) especially when the worry and excitement bring on diarrhoea

MEDICINE	AILMENT/CONDITION	SYMPTOMS WORSEN/IMPROVE	NOTES
ARSEN. ALB. (*Arsenicum album*)	*Anxiety* (and great fear) Will also help: restlessness; burning pains; dry and burning throat; burning pain in the stomach; excessive thirst but with the desire to sip only, little and often; food poisoning; inability to bear the sight or smell of food; difficult breathing with the need to sit or bend forward	*Worsen* after midnight; between 1 and 2 pm; at the coast; from cold and wet weather; *improve* by keeping warm, with cool air round the head	Suited to excessively tidy, fussy and precise individuals who feel the cold
BRYONIA (*Bryonia alba*)	*Irritability* Will also help: chestiness – colds often go down into the chest; dryness; dry, painful cough, often violent; dry lips; excessive thirst,	*Worsen* from any movement; from warmth; *improve* from cold food and drinks; from pressure (except on the abdomen); from rest;	Suited to individuals with dark hair and complexion who may be subject to rheumatism or bilious attacks

	especially for cold drinks; food lies like a stone in the stomach which is too painful to touch; diarrhoea after eating over-ripe fruit	while lying on the painful side	
CALC. CARB. (*Calcarea carbonica*)	*Excessive appetite and fat* *Breast tenderness* Will also help: craving for eggs and sweets; aversion to milk; may feel generally better when constipated; tendency to feel the cold and to catch cold easily; profuse periods in young girls	*Worsen* from cold; in damp weather; at night; from standing; at full moon; *improve* in dry weather; from warmth (avoid sun); while lying on the painful side	Suited to quiet, shy, sensitive people who are subject to depression; who often have a feeling of being looked at by everyone and a fear of being laughed at and are embarrassed when entering a room full of strangers

MEDICINE	AILMENT/CONDITION	SYMPTOMS WORSEN/IMPROVE	NOTES
CALC. PHOS. (*Calcarea phosphorica*)	*Periods too early and excessive* Will also help: headache from change of weather; severe stomach pain after eating; fractures which are slow to heal; rheumatic pain following exposure to draughts; acne	*Worsen* from any change in the weather	Suited to individuals who tend to be absent-minded and touchy
EUPHRASIA (*Euphrasia officinalis*)	*Headaches* Will also help: colds with watering eyes and streaming nose; inflamed eyes which sting and burn; conjunctivitis; inability to bear bright light; hay fever; first stage of measles	*Worsen* in the evening; in bed; when indoors; from warmth; in bright light; *improve* in dim light or darkness; from cold applications	

FERR. PHOS. (*Ferrum phosphoricum*)	*Excessive appetite* (varies greatly from that insatiable hunger to total loss of appetite) Will also help: fear of crowds, of impending misfortune, of death; dizziness from congestion to parts of the head; suitable for first stage of acute inflammation and early colds, especially when without very definite symptoms; over-excitability and talkativeness	*Worsen* at night; from cold; from touch; *improve* in summer; from warmth; from cold applications; while slowly walking around	Suited to people who are pale and of a delicate physique, who flush easily on exertion or with a slight rise in temperature. They are quick to anger, prefer to be left alone, are often intolerant of noise and generally suffer from a feeling of inadequacy

MEDICINE	AILMENT/CONDITION	SYMPTOMS WORSEN/IMPROVE	NOTES
GRAPHITES (Graphites)	*Excess fat* Will also help: unhealthy skin; cracked, weeping eczema; tendency for injuries to suppurate; cracked finger-tips; constipation; strange symptom of being able to hear better in noisy situations; sensation of cobwebs on the face	*Worsen* at night; during and after periods; *improve* in the dark; from wrapping up	Suited to individuals who are by nature extremely cautious and who find difficulty in making decisions
IGNATIA (*Ignatia amara*)	*Depression/Piercing headache* Will also help: mental shock; fright; prolonged grief; piles which protrude easily, with stitching pains in the rectum, and which are better while walking;		Suited to emotional and sensitive people who are easily moved to tears and who prefer to be left alone

sore throat relieved by swallowing; dislike of tobacco smoke

KALI. BICH. (*Kalium bichromicum*)	*Migraine* (blurred vision before headache) Will also help: complaints brought on by a change to hot weather; catarrh with a stringy discharge; sinus troubles; hard cough with stringy sputum; sore throat; pains moving rapidly from place to place; nausea and vomiting after alcohol	*Worsen* in the morning; from alcohol; during hot weather; *improve* from heat

MEDICINE	AILMENT/CONDITION	SYMPTOMS WORSEN/IMPROVE	NOTES
KALI. PHOS. (*Kalium phosphoricum*)	*Headache* (with humming in the ears following mental effort) Will also help: mental tiredness from overwork; nervous exhaustion; nervous indigestion; indigestion following a 'working lunch'; exhaustion following long periods of preparation for examinations; loss of voice or hoarseness after over-exertion and constant use of the voice; giddiness from exhaustion and weakness; bad breath; dry tongue in the morning	*Worsen* from noise; from mental exertion; *improve* during gentle movement; from warmth; after nourishment	Suited to shy individuals with a poor memory

LYCOPODIUM (Lycopodium clavatum)	Sugar and carbohydrate cravings	Worsen (symptoms	Suited to people who
	Excessive appetite (even at night but which is easily satisfied)	mostly on the right side) between 4 and 6 pm; in stuffy rooms; from cold; from noise; *improve* after warm drinks; on loosening clothing around the abdomen; in fresh air	are intense, conscientious and of keen intellect but who nevertheless feel insecure. They cannot endure contradiction, but seek argument. Often they are of pale complexion with thin, deep furrows
	Will also help: irritability; dislike of exercise; fear of failure; preference to be alone (but with somebody near); craving for sweet foods even though they cause indigestion; coldness in one foot (usually the right) while the other is warm; pains which go from left to right		

MEDICINE	AILMENT/CONDITION	SYMPTOMS WORSEN/IMPROVE	NOTES
NAT. MUR. (*Natrium muriaticum*)	*Migraine/Headaches* (hammering headache preceded by misty vision or zig-zag lights) Will also help: sneezy colds; nose running like a tap (treat quickly at the onset); sinus troubles; eczema at the borders of the hair; herpes of lips; use of a lot of salt on food; continuous thirst; dislike of bread; exhaustion	*Worsen* in mid-morning; near the coast; while lying down; *improve* in the open air; while lying on the right side; with cold bathing	Suited to those of a pale complexion and oily skin who tend to feel insecure, worry about the future and are easily moved to tears. They are irritable and quarrelsome, do not wish to be ignored but dislike consolation.
NUX VOM. (*Nux vomica*)	*Irritability* Will also help: nervousness; nervous indigestion; over-sensitivity to noise, odours, light, music;	*Worsen* between 3 and 4 am; from cold; *improve* in the evening; from being covered; from warmth	Suited to thin dark people who are inclined to be impatient and irritable

trifling ailments seeming unbearable; ill-effects of over-eating or drinking; early morning liverishness; fussiness about food, liking for fatty foods; indigestion; dislike of coffee and tobacco smoke; pain, like a stone in the stomach, two to three hours after eating; constipation, with ineffectual urging; itching piles; stuffy colds; raw throat

MEDICINE	AILMENT/CONDITION	SYMPTOMS WORSEN/IMPROVE	NOTES
PULSATILLA (*pulsatilla nigricans*)	*Periods suppressed, delayed, or scanty yet protracted* *Excess fat* Will also help: catarrh (yellow-green thick discharge); styes (especially on upper lids); mumps; measles; change of life; aversion to fat or greasy food; absence of thirst (even in fever) though the mouth may be dry; rapid change in symptoms – from feeling well to feeling miserable; rapidly shifting pains	*Worsen* in the evening; from heat; after eating rich foods; from sudden chilling; *improve* in the open air; from cold applications; after cold food and drinks; while lying on the painful side	Suited to females with fair hair, blue eyes and fair or pale complexion (often with pink patches). They are affectionate, easily moved to laughter or tears, shy, never obstinate but like and seek sympathy. They are sensitive to reprimand and tend to put on fat easily. They dislike extremes of weather.
SEPIA (Sepia)	*Depression/Periods suppressed or delayed*	*Worsen* in the afternoon and evening; from cold;	Suited to thin dark-haired people of

	Will also help	Worse / Improve	Suited to
	great fear of injections; indifference to loved ones; sadness and fear of being left alone; yellowness – especially of the face, with a saddle across the nose; faint 'all-gone' sensation in the middle of the morning; morning sickness in pregnancy; sensitivity to the cold; periods suppressed or delayed; change of life	before thunder; from tobacco smoke; *improve* in a warm bed; from hot applications	below average height. They are easily depressed (particularly women), and are likely to harbour real or imaginary fears. They have little interest in work or recreation
SULPHUR (Sulphur)	*Anxiety* Will also help: unhealthy looking skin; tendency to skin diseases; body odour; tendency to sweat easily; orifices of body too red (e.g. lips); burning pains; feet needing to be placed	*Worsen* from cold; from dampness; at the coast; *improve* from warmth; in fresh air	Suited to deep-thinking people who have a nervous yet independent nature

Continued over page

MEDICINE	AILMENT/CONDITION	SYMPTOMS WORSEN/IMPROVE	NOTES
	outside the bedclothes to cool; burning and itching piles; itching skin — scratching pleasurable but results in burning; mid-morning hunger; large appetite for highly seasoned, spicy and fatty foods; liking for sweets; aggravation from milk; diarrhoea; constipation, with large painful stools; lack of energy (regained quickly at the prospect of pleasurable activity); tendency to become exhausted quickly, perhaps fainting; tendency to catch cold easily, which often goes into the chest; asthma		

CHAPTER EIGHT

Herbalism and Herbal Remedies

The use of herbal medicine in Britain dates back to pre-Roman times. The Druid priest-healers, as well as being extremely skilled in the use of herbal remedies, believed that the moon exerted a powerful cyclical influence on both man and plant. Henry VIII was an enthusiastic user of herbal treatments and went so far as to devise his own recipes. In fact, herbalists today are still protected by a Royal Charter dating back to the time of his reign.

Herbal recipes were passed down the generations, and in the seventeenth century a woman knew exactly which herb was beneficial for a variety of ailments. Nowadays most of us wouldn't know a comfrey plant if it was staring us in the face. If we did recognize it, I doubt that many of us would know what to do with it!

At the start of this century the progress of science, plus the business and commercial activities of pharmaceutical companies, drove herbalism practically out of existence with just a few people struggling to keep knowledge of herbal remedies alive.

However the situation now seems to be changing, as we have become increasingly disillusioned with so-called safe drugs.

The main principle to remember with herbalism is that the *whole* plant is used in medications, whereas pharmaceutical companies working with plants only extract a *part*. As every plant contains substances which have opposing and balancing effects on the body, it is the herbalist's view that the use of the whole plant avoids many of the dangers that can occur when just one part is isolated.

Let us take an example of a common drug to illustrate this point. Willow (*Salix alba*) has been used for centuries as a remedy for aches, pains and fevers. During this century salicin was isolated from the plant; from salicin came salicylic acid, and from these two derivatives a substance called acetylsalicylic acid – more usually known as aspirin. Common side-effects of this drug are nausea, vomiting, heartburn and indigestion, with prolonged use at times causing kidney damage.

What begins as a completely natural substance ends up in drug form far removed from anything that can be described in these terms. Drug companies shroud the entire manufacturing process under patent law, so there is no way of knowing exactly how a particular drug is made. It is not that herbal medicines should be underestimated – they can be extremely potent, which is where a trained medical herbalist comes in. Herbs are very valuable for use in the home, but unless you are skilled they will not answer all your medical needs.

Primitive peoples, living thousands of miles apart, have used an infusion of *Hibiscus rosa sinensis* for menstrual problems and also to regulate fertility. In Mexico, Zoapatl (*Montanor tormentosa*) is used widely for menstrual problems. Here in the UK things are different and we do not use herbal remedies for regulating the menstrual cycle; yet some of them work extremely well, bringing quick relief – safely.

One which needs a special mention and is readily available in the UK is Agnus Castus, a herbal remedy which is particularly effective in reducing PMT symptoms. It is the fruit from the Chaste Tree, or Monk's Pepper, and is grown in North Africa. The department of gynaecology of the University of Gottingen conducted a number of experiments with Agnus Castus and although hormones were not found within the fruit, the volatile oil appears to influence the pituitary gland and increases the output of certain hormones which regulate the function of the corpus luteum. (The latter produces oestrogen and progesterone during the menstrual cycle.) In short, Agnus Castus encourages the glandular system to produce its own hormones. It is taken in tablet form, 2 tablets three times a day after food. Women have reported very good results after taking this remedy, such as the easing of period pains, also the reduction of depression, irritability, tension, mood swings and migraine-type headaches. Some women found that all their symptoms went when taking this particular remedy, so it is well worth a try.

There are a number of other herbs which work well for certain PMT symptoms, and these are best bought in dried form. Make sure they are kept in cool conditions in light-proof containers, as both light and heat can destroy the vital properties of the herbs.

Should you think of growing your own herbs, let me warn you that this can be fraught with difficulties. You will have to make sure your plants are not contaminated with lead pollution from traffic and are kept well clear of any chemical sprays. To dry out herbs is not a simple task, as you could well destroy the volatile oils. Take the easy way out and buy what you need, preferably from a specialist shop with a high turnover so that you can be sure of top quality, well-kept herbs.

Dried herbs can be taken in two ways – as infusions and decoctions.

Infusions These are made by steeping the leafy and flowering parts of the plant. Put one to three teaspoons in a thermos flask with one cup of boiling water. Close the thermos immediately to keep in the steam and stop the essential oils from disappearing.

Decoctions These are made from the roots and bark of the plant. Place one ounce of your chosen remedy in one pint of water and simmer in a saucepan (*not aluminium*) with the lid on for ten to fifteen minutes.

Your herbal remedy can be taken either hot or cold. When taking a remedy as a diuretic to ease water retention, wait for it to cool down – it works better this way.

I should warn you now that many herbal remedies taste bitter, so you must either grin and bear it, or add a little honey if you cannot!

Herbal Remedies For PMT Symptoms

Many herbs have more than one use, so look up your symptoms and choose one of the herbs listed. If your selected remedy is not successful, try an alternative – this way you will find out which is the most effective for you. If you think any remedy is not agreeing with you, stop taking it immediately. This does not mean that herbal remedies are not for you, merely that you need either to select a different one or go to a qualified medical herbalist for advice.

SYMPTOM	HERBAL REMEDY	NOTES
FLUID RETENTION	Couch grass (*Agropyron repens*)	Can also be taken for cystitis.
	Dandelion leaf (*Taraxacum officinale*)	Also known as 'Pis-en-lit'! It has a strong diuretic action and is rich in potassium, therefore there is no need to take a potassium supplement as is the case with most drug diuretics. Probably the best remedy for fluid retention.
	Vervain (*Verbena officinalis*)	This diuretic can also ease painful periods and migraine attacks.
		Do not boil these herbs, and take the remedy cold. The diuretic action is better when the herb is left to cool.

SYMPTOM	HERBAL REMEDY	NOTES
HEADACHE	Catmint (*Nepeta cataria*)	Do not boil this remedy.
	Lavender (*Lavandula vera*)	Rub a little lavender oil into the temples, but not too much as it's very strong. A couple of drops is adequate.
	Meadowsweet (*Filipendula ulmaria*)	This has many of the properties of aspirin with none of the side-effects.
	Rosemary (*Rosmarinus officinalis*)	The leaves can be taken as an infusion, or rosemary oil can be rubbed gently into the temples. It is also an anti-depressant.
	Valerian (*Valeriana officinalis*)	*Warning* Use only small doses, as this is a powerful sedative and does not agree with everyone. Best taken in tablet form if in any doubt. Can also be used for reducing tension and insomnia.

SYMPTOM	HERBAL REMEDY	NOTES
MIGRAINE	Feverfew (*Chrysanthemum parthenium*)	Take as an infusion, or the fresh leaves can be put in a sandwich to disguise the bitter taste.
	Vervain (*Verbena officinalis*)	Take as an infusion.
INSOMNIA	Chamomile (*Anthemis nobilis*)	This is a famous herbal remedy, which as well as assisting sleep has a calming effect on the nervous system.
	Limeflowers (*Tilia*)	Drink just before you go to bed.
	Valerian (*Valeriana officinalis*)	*See* Headache for warning on use.
DEPRESSION	Lemon balm (*Melissa officinalis*)	(Also relieves tension)
	Rosemary (*Rosmarinus officinalis*)	These remedies can be taken as an infusion throughout the day.
	St John's wort (*Hypericum perforatum*)	

SYMPTOM	HERBAL REMEDY	NOTES
TENSION	Lemon balm (*Melissa officinalis*)	*See* Depression
	Motherwort (*Leonurus cardiaca*)	This is a traditional remedy for women's ailments, also relieving period pains.
	Sage leaves (*Saliva officinalis*)	The Chinese use sage leaves in place of tea. This has a soothing and calming effect, as well as being an excellent tonic if you are feeling low.
	Valerian (*Valeriana officinalis*)	*See* Headache for warning on use.
SICKNESS AND NAUSEA	Lavender (*Lavandula vera*)	Drink as an infusion until sickness goes.
	Raspberry leaves (*Rubus idaens*)	Also good for heavy periods.
GENERAL HEALTH TONICS	Licorice (*Glycyrrhiza glabra*)	In Chinese herbal medicine this has been used as a very effective tonic for women. You can put licorice with more bitter-tasting remedies, as it is quite sweet to taste.

SYMPTOM	HERBAL REMEDY	NOTES
	Nettle (*Urtica dioica*)	This remedy is particularly rich in minerals. The new green shoots of the plant can be eaten in soups or used as a vegetable. (Wear gloves when harvesting!)
	Sage leaves (*Saliva officinalis*)	*See* Tension
	Sqawvine (*Mitchella ripens*)	*See* Painful and scanty periods
PAINFUL PERIODS Although not strictly related to PMT, I am including the following list of herbs which can be helpful with various problems connected with menstruation.	Marigold flowers (*Calendula officinalis*) Motherwort (*Leonurus cardiaca*) Sqawvine (*Mitchella ripens*) Vervain (*Verbena officinalis*)	All of the following remedies can be taken as infusions.
HEAVY PERIODS	Raspberry leaves (*Rubus idaens*)	Reduces the menstrual flow without stopping it.

SYMPTOM	HERBAL REMEDY	NOTES
IRREGULAR PERIODS	Rosemary (*Rosmarinus officinalis*)	
	St John's wort (*Hypericum perforatum*)	
SCANTY PERIODS	Sqawvine (*Mitchella ripens*)	

CHAPTER NINE

Stress and Strain

First of all, what exactly is stress? It is the way in which we as individuals respond to challenging situations. For instance, you are asked to make a speech and on comes an attack of 'nerves'. What is happening to cause these feelings? Your apprehension at having to stand up before a group of people causes your brain to signal for extra adrenalin, which in turn causes an increase in your heartbeat, blood pressure and breathing rate. This is to prepare you for action.

Once the first few minutes of your performance have passed, the body still has to function at a higher level until the speech is over. Most of us spend the majority of the day in this second phase, which helps us to cope with everyday living. It is also a phase that brings with it creativity and a feeling of well-being.

Finally there can be a stage which is dangerous, and this comes when the body cannot cope and starts to wear out; at this point symptoms of fatigue and illnesses occur, and stress can show in many ways. Depression, anxiety, irritability, fear and aggression can all be signs. Further indications may be an overall tenseness of the body, shown in poor posture, nervous habits and up-tight facial expressions. When the body is not functioning efficiently, the immune system starts to fail and we become vulnerable to illness.

Stress occurs every day of our lives and a certain amount is essential to our well-being. With no stress at all, our bodies would collapse, our functions deteriorate and our lives become meaningless. Some stress, then, is necessary for us to function as physical beings, but for the most part we are unaware of it.

We experience many different types of stress all the time.

Excitement and happiness (a first job or wedding day) can be labelled 'stress', just as much as shock and unhappiness (redundancy or divorce). There are unavoidable causes of stress – earthquakes, for example – as well as those such as rush-hour travelling which we can try to change. Stress can occur from events in the outside world as well as from internal differences and individuals vary in their reactions to it; like thresholds of pain, some can tolerate vast amounts of excitement and difficulties, whilst others feel the impact much earlier. All of us have our own levels of stress which we find acceptable and tolerable, but for each of us there comes a point beyond which we cannot cope. For some, it might be the umpteenth time the toothpaste top is left off or the cupboard door not closed; for others, the bankruptcy of a company could be the 'last straw'. We start questioning stress only when it seems to be adversely affecting our lives – harming, upsetting or damaging us.

Severe trauma can disrupt the menstrual cycle. For example, painful periods and severe pelvic pain can be the direct result of going through a divorce. Emotional stress can also cause weight gain; many women turn for comfort to food in the form of cream cakes, biscuits and chocolate. A raw carrot or stick of celery just doesn't have the same effect!

Whereas major stresses in life can cause the body to be vulnerable to ill-health, minor stresses cause tension which in turn localizes in various areas. Examples are headache, eye strain, pains in the shoulders, neck and throat, lower back, stomach and digestive system.

These minor stresses and their physical manifestations may well play a part in your PMT symptoms. To be able to decide whether stress is an important factor for you, the following Stress Check List should help to highlight areas of stress in your life now. The Check List considers a variety of aspects of living which demand *some* stress – family, work, social, personal, environment. Opposite each item on the list, put *a tick* (✓) in one of the three columns to show whether this is a major, minor or no-stress factor for you.

Stress Check List

POSSIBLE STRESS	MAJOR STRESS	MINOR STRESS	NO STRESS
Daily childcare			—
Dependent relatives			—
Parental pressure			—
Troublesome in-laws			—
Demanding teenagers			—
Children leaving home			—
Partner's frequent absence			—
Sole responsibility for family			—
Marriage worries			—
Home/work conflicts		✓	
Inability to get a job			—
Too little partner/family support		✓	
Lack of mental stimulation			—
Frustrated ambitions		✓	
Physical overwork	✓	✓	
Boring, repetitive work			—
Difficulties with people at work			—
'Rat-race' lifestyle		✓	
Can't delegate			—
Feeling trapped		✓	
Feeling misunderstood		✓	
Feeling taken for granted, useless		✓	
Feeling lonely, isolated			—
Feeling rusty, out of touch			—
No time for myself			—
Getting a raw deal from everyone			—
Giving in to people too much			—
Missing fun, excitement		✓	
Feeling angry, afraid			—

11/86

Severe PMT - off work for first time with this.

POSSIBLE STRESS	MAJOR STRESS	MINOR STRESS	NO STRESS
Newly single again			✓
No special close friend			✓
Away from home for the first time			✓
Missing family, friends – isolated			✓
Feeling fat, ugly		✓	✓
Needing romance			✓
Needing hobbies, interests			✓
Too few social opportunities		✓	✓
Feeling shy, lacking confidence			✓
Monotonous evenings, weekends		✓	
Unpleasant living location *weather*	✓		
Noisy neighbours			✓
Rush hour travelling			✓
Pressure from TV/radio/media			✓
Traffic disturbance			✓
Aircraft noise			✓
Long distance to shops, transport		✓	
Unhappy with accommodation		✓	

OTHER STRESSES IN MY LIFE:
Have there been any *major* changes in your life over the past six months? Think of happy as well as sad events and write details of recent life changes here:

– Changes at work = new boss
                   = new class

+ Building house – a relief to start

– No holidays – not properly anyway

+ Mod trip to Edin.

– Jealousy

– Consistent bad weather

Coping Strategies Profile – How Do You Cope?

How do *you* cope with the stresses and strains of living? We have many individual reactions to happiness and sadness, and respond to different types of stress in unique ways. If the boss gets you down or the toddlers whine constantly, are you the patient angel or a quick-draw reacter? Often the world expects women to be assertive yet unruffled, imaginative yet conforming, tranquil yet uninhibited – there seems no perfect formula!

There are *no* right or wrong answers to this Profile, which seeks to help increase your awareness of ways of coping in general with emergencies, crisis, decision and action points. You can also use this chart to identify how you cope with each individual stress you have ticked in the Stress Check List on pp. 92–3. Put a ring around ONE of the numbers in between the following adjectives according to how well you think each pair describes your usual coping strategy. Use the numbers as follows:

1 This is the way I *always* cope
2 This is the way I *sometimes* cope
3 This is the way I *rarely* cope
4 I'm unsure whether I cope either way

Assertive	1 2 ③ 4 3 2 1	Disregarding
Wavering	1 2 ③ 4 3 2 1	Confident
Unruffled	1 2 3 4 ③ 2 1	Easily upset
Slow	1 2 3 4 ③ 2 1	Quick
Prudent	1 2 3 ④ 3 2 1	Impulsive
Casual	1 2 3 4 ② 2 1	Formal
Shy	1 2 ③ 4 3 2 1	Uninhibited
No nonsense	1 2 3 4 3 ② 1	Tender
Trusting	1 2 3 4 3 ② 1	Suspicious
Practical	1 ② 3 4 3 2 1	Imaginative
Forthright	1 2 3 4 ③ 2 1	Shrewd
Experimental	1 2 3 4 ③ 2 1	Cautious
Dependent	1 2 3 ④ 3 2 1	Independent
Socially precise	1 2 ③ 4 3 2 1	Impetuous
Tense	1 ② 3 4 3 2 1	Tranquil
Superior	1 2 ③ 4 3 2 1	Inferior

Competitive	1 2 3 4 3 ②1	Co-operative
Active	1 2 3 ④ 3 2 1	Passive
Indifferent	1 2 3 ④ 3 2 1	Curious
Safe	1 ② 3 4 3 2 1	Risky
Aggressive	1 2 3 4 ③ 2 1	Afraid
Cheerful	1 2 3 4 ③ 2 1	Complaining
Gossipy	1 2 3 4 ③ 2 1	Tactful
Disapproving	1 2 3 4 ③ 2 1	Accepting
Competent	1 ② 3 4 3 2 1	Incapable

After you have finished answering, you might like to join all the circled numbers down with a line. This line will indicate the main direction of your responses to obtain a Profile of your usual Coping Strategy. If you have a line swinging across lots of 1s, this can show a very strong Profile, sometimes extreme. On the other hand, if there are many 4s, this might suggest somewhat uncertain ways of coping. Most people will find a mixed or varied Profile.

Stress Check List and Coping Strategies Profile reproduced by kind permission of Linda R. Greenbury, of the Career Development Centre 4 Women (CDC4W)

CHAPTER TEN

Relaxation, Acupressure Techniques and Exercise

Relaxation

The most difficult thing to do when you are worried, anxious and under strain is to relax. Stress causes many symptoms such as headaches, stiffness of joints, tenseness of the body, back pain, palpitations, sweating, fatigue and lethargy. Depending on your temperament, it can cause outward signs of irritability, anger and aggression to the other extreme of wanting to close the curtains, bolt the door and remain hidden from the world.

Often there is a sense of isolation when we go through anything we perceive as being a major stress. Who can we turn to for help? There are organizations which have counsellors to aid if you are feeling depressed and despairing, but by far the best place to turn to is your family and close friends; learn to express your feelings and whilst they may not be able to solve your problems they can certainly give love and support whilst you sort yourself out. Sometimes however this is not possible. Perhaps your family members live too far away – or the very problems you are trying to overcome may be family orientated. Maybe you even feel, for whatever reason, that you haven't a friend you can turn to. In this case look up the address of a relaxation class, or become involved in something which interests you. When you meet people with similar interests, you have something in common from the start; that will create a bond which could lead to new friendships. It is very important to reduce any feelings of isolation when times are tough. Ultimately we are responsible for ourselves and must learn to control any situations which cause stress.

Suppose there are a number of problematical areas in your life? One of the worst things to do is to attempt to solve them all overnight. Decide which situation can be resolved fairly easily, get on with it and leave the more difficult decisions to a later date. Eventually your life will become easier, but take everything in stages. We all need an inner strength to survive life's hassles, and one of the best ways is through relaxation: a time of peace set aside just for you, with no outside interference, when you can concentrate on easing your mind and body. One of the best ways I found was something I called my 'total relaxation routine'. I passed this on to a number of women who said they also found it helpful.

TOTAL RELAXATION ROUTINE

Plan for at least one – or better still, two – periods of time during your waking hours when you can arrange not to be disturbed. Tell everyone to keep away for about half an hour; take the 'phone off the hook, jam the doorbell so that it won't ring during your relaxation period; even lock the door to your room if necessary! Obviously the ideal place to relax is at home, but I know of a woman who carried out her routine in a store-room at work during her lunchtime period. If you don't fancy that type of environment, then home is the place for you! Draw the curtains, dim the lights (or use candlelight), make sure your clothing is loose and comfortable and put on some music. If you are feeling emotional, don't play a sad love song or you will be in tears before you even begin. On the other hand, if you're feeling uptight or in a real rage, I would suggest you steer clear of Tchaikovsky's '1812' Overture or at the first thunder of the cannon you'll be up to kick the furniture or worse! Select something instrumental which is gentle to the ears and play at a low volume! If your musical taste doesn't run to this type of music, then buy a tape of relaxation music; these are now widely available. The scene is set and it's time to begin.

Either sit on a chair with your legs raised on a stool to hip level, or lie flat on the floor. Make yourself as comfortable as you can and close your eyes. Take in a slow deep breath, hold it for about three seconds, then let it out slowly. Repeat this half a dozen times and you will begin to feel a calming sensation.

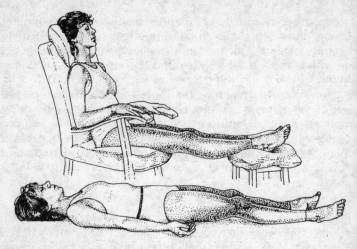

Figure 5: Total Relaxation Routine

Now you are going to start relaxing your body, by concentrating your mind and visualizing all the tension flowing out of each part. Begin with your toes, moving to the ankles and then upwards to your calves, knees, thighs and hips. Take plenty of time and don't move on to the next part of your body until you can mentally imagine the tension receding from the area you're working on. When your legs are feeling heavy, move to your hands – concentrating on letting the tension go – and then slowly to the wrists, elbows, lower and upper arms. Unhurriedly change your thoughts to the hip area, then gradually upwards to the abdomen, chest, shoulders and neck. By now you will be much calmer and your body will be feeling heavy. Still taking plenty of time, move to your face; you will find that, compared with your body, it seems to be in a vice-like grip. Move up the chin, to the mouth, lips, cheeks, eyes and forehead. The face muscles will relax as you imagine all that tension going. Remain as you are for five to ten minutes but don't let your mind wander – keep your concentration directed on this soothing feeling of total relaxation. You may want to fall asleep, which is no bad thing if you have the time. Otherwise, arrange for your alarm clock to ring softly after about thirty minutes. I use my cooker timer, which has a gentle ping!

When you move, don't immediately jump into action. Move gently and slowly. Sit still for a couple of minutes, then go and make yourself a warm drink and take the time to enjoy it. You deserve it!

You may need to practise this routine a number of times before you get to the stage of feeling totally relaxed. Don't give up! One very good time to practise is when you go to bed. This is a programme which will give complete relaxation to mind and body, as well as soothing and resting all the nerves and muscles.

Acupressure

This is another form of relaxation which you can do by yourself easily, and is an offshoot from acupuncture. Oriental medicine is based on the belief that there is a life energy called Chi, and that health is only possible when the Chi is flowing throughout the body in sufficient quantities. This life energy energizes all the cells and tissues of the body. Acupuncture treats the patient as a whole – mind, body and spirit – but most of all it is a preventive medicine. In fact in ancient times, the mandarins had a great scheme which I wish we could follow today – they paid their physicians to keep them in good health and stopped all payments when they fell ill! The life energy Chi is thought to be distributed throughout the body in channels called meridians, which flow deep into the body and surface on the skin. The places where they surface are known as the acupuncture points and it is at these points that the acupuncturist inserts needles which stimulate the flow of energy through the body.

Acupressure is a development from acupuncture and uses the same points by means of the fingers and thumbs instead of needles. Its main use is to correct the imbalances in the nervous system; stimulation of certain points can be very beneficial for certain PMT symptoms.

The following acupressure exercises should not be used if you are pregnant or have serious heart or circulatory problems, nor in the case of severe and continuous fatigue.

HOW TO USE ACUPRESSURE

Set aside plenty of time for the exercises and make sure you will not be disturbed. Wear loose clothing and either sit or lie down in a comfortable position. If you wish you can have a friend massage the various points for you, or you can do it yourself.

Use either the tips or balls of the fingers, with your nails trimmed to avoid bruising. Begin by putting the pad of your finger on the point indicated, making sure the finger does not wander off the position whilst applying massage. You need to sustain pressure on the point. If your finger starts to get tired, then ease off, relax and start again.

The healing points are activated as follows: (a) acute complaints – light circular massage for up to five minutes; (b) chronic complaints – medium to strong massage for up to one minute, several times per day.

HOW TO FIND THE ACUPRESSURE POINT

The drawings on pp. 102–3 will help you to find the point, but since we are all different the exact position changes with the individual. Normally when you find the right spot you will feel it to be either tender or painful.

Exercise 1: (Fig. 6) *Frontal headache*. Place the balls of your thumbs on either side of your head and massage lightly, both sides at the same time. You may find it more beneficial if your eyes are closed.

Exercise 2: (Fig. 7) *Migraine-type headache*. Place the ball of your first finger on your other hand as shown, with the ball of your thumb on the underneath. Use light pressure for up to five minutes.

Exercise 3: (Fig. 8) *Headache at the back of the head*. Place the first fingers of both hands, or the thumbs, at the base of the skull. Each finger should be approximately one inch to one side of the centre of your neck, just below the skull bone. Use strong pressure on both sides at the same time.

Exercise 4 (Fig. 9) *Anxiety*. The position of this point is found by firstly bringing your finger to a position 2¾ inches down from the knee, then moving to the side of the leg in a straight vertical line to a position approximately a third of the way back from the front of the leg. Using the pads of the fingers, lightly massage both sides at the same time for up to five minutes.

Exercise 5 (Fig. 10) *Tension*. Place your fingers as shown, with thumbs on the front of your neck. The position of the fingers should be half-way between the top of your shoulders and the beginning of your collar-bone. Start by lightly massaging the points on both sides between your thumbs and fingers, gradually increasing to stronger pressure.

Exercise 6 (Fig. 11) *Fatigue*. This massage should be done with your thumbnail placed in the crease of the top joint of the little finger. Use strong massage for up to five minutes. This can be repeated hourly if required.

Exercise 7 (Fig. 12) *Weight reduction*. The point to find is half-way down the upper portion of your arm – move to the side of the arm vertically and massage at the centre of the side. Using the ball of your finger, apply light pressure for up to a minute. This is a point which reduces the appetite and slows down metabolism.

Exercise 8 (Fig. 13) *Lack of sleep or disturbed sleep*. Put your thumb behind the lobe of your ear, with the ball of your finger on the front of the lobe. Using light pressure, massage the lobe; your finger should move more quickly than your thumb. Continue for up to five minutes.

OTHER METHODS OF RELAXATION
There are many paths to choose from on your road to relaxation, and the choice as to which one you practise is personal to you. Below is a brief description of various relaxation methods; addresses to contact are listed in Chapter 12.

Yoga. Yoga concentrates on three main areas – posture, breathing and meditation. There are many types of yoga, but normally the emphasis at the start of all courses is to achieve mind control. After you have learnt the exercises you can continue using them by yourself at home.

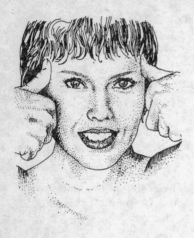

Figure 6: Frontal Headache

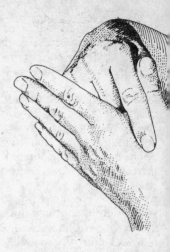

Figure 7: Migraine-type Headac

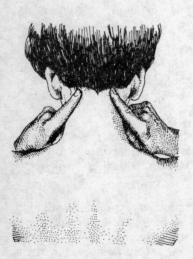

Figure 8: Headache At Back of Head

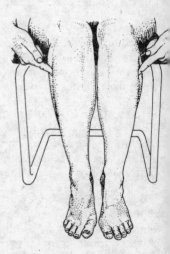

Figure 9: Anxiety

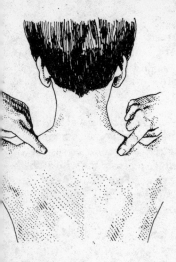

Figure 10: Tension

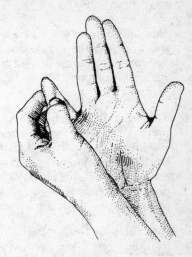

Figure 11: Fatigue

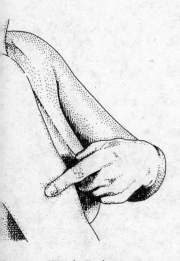

Figure 12: Weight Reduction

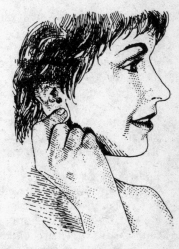

Figure 13: Lack Of Sleep

Shiatsu. Shiatsu is a Japanese word meaning 'finger pressure' and was originally the Japanese form of Chinese acupressure. It has developed into a therapy of its own, but basically shiatsu and acupressure (which I have dealt with earlier in this chapter) are very much the same thing.

The Alexander principle. This is basically a therapy which aims to prevent and treat a wide variety of problems by changing the posture of the individual. One of the benefits this system of treatment seems to bring in its wake is relief from the strain which can be caused by the body not being aligned correctly. As it is not possible to teach yourself the Alexander principle, you will need to go to classes if you are interested.

Reflexology. It seems possible that a form of reflexology was used in China over 5,000 years ago. A reflexologist works with ten channels (energy zones) all of which begin or end in the toes. Working with the feet, a trained practitioner can tell which channels are blocked. By massaging the correct point of the foot, using the techniques of shiatsu, it is possible to restore the correct balance of energy in the body. Amongst other things, this therapy is supposed to relax both body and mind.

Applied kinesiology ('Touch for Health'). This is based on special muscle-testing techniques through which weaknesses in the body can be identified and treated; the end result is a balanced energy system running through the body. Kinesiology has certain similarities to the chiropractic and massage approaches. It also shares the same philosophy as acupuncture and shiatsu – it works on the energy fields in the body. Kinesiology is not a self-help method of treatment; you will need to go to a professional. However, 'Touch for Health' can be taught and is basically the art of using touch as a means to transmit healing forces.

Body massage. You can easily teach yourself the art of massage through any one of the excellent books available on the subject. You will need to bribe a relative or friend to give you a massage – but you, of course, will offer a reciprocal favour!! Aromatic oils can be used, which are marvellous for relaxation and tension as well as leaving a beautiful lingering perfume in the air.

Any activity which takes your mind off your troubles is a good way to relax. Take up a new hobby, play an instrument, read an absorbing book. If you live on your own, invite friends in for decaffeinated coffee! If on the other hand you are surrounded by a demanding family, get out of the house for a while and take the dog for a walk. Dogs are great company and will listen to all your hard luck stories and not answer back! If you don't own a dog – borrow one!

Exercise

All forms of exercise are beneficial to health, provided you are under the care of qualified teachers and do not end up with injuries. If you are a sports-orientated person, there is no need for me to tell you what to do. However, I am thinking particularly of all those who, like me, have to make a concerted effort to do any type of exercise and feel that if it can be avoided altogether so much the better!! So many of the sports require special clothing and equipment; the cost of all the gear would pay for a week's holiday in the sunnier parts of the continent! So here's my answer to the keep-fit boom, which will cost you nothing provided you have a comfortable pair of shoes. It is safe, painless and you can do it for a lifetime – Walking!

When exercise was originally considered scientifically it was walking which was studied. In the early fifties, Professor J. N. Morris found that fatal heart attacks were less likely for people who walked rather than sat at their jobs. In the eighties investigations carried out at the Oshsner Clinic in New Orleans concluded that moderate exercise, such as walking, could help those who had suffered a heart attack as well as those 'at risk'. Brisk walking was found to be helpful in lowering high blood pressure, as well as increasing the blood levels of high-density lipoprotein cholesterol materials which help to prevent heart attacks.

Dr Grant Gwinup of the University of California gave the following advice to a group of obese women who had been unable to lose weight by dieting:

- Don't try to diet

- Take a daily walk
- Gradually increase the time and distance

The women gradually increased to a daily walk of 30 minutes, and during the following year lost an average of twenty-two pounds.

Further research in America has shown the following:

- Daily exercise such as a 45-minute brisk walk can mean a loss of twenty to thirty pounds of fat within a year.
- Walking within two to three hours of eating burns off more calories than exercising on an empty stomach.
- The mind works better when the body is in motion.
- Physical activity can help to improve decision-making.
- Walking is more effective than tranquillizers in reducing muscular tension and anxiety.
- A major cause of adult-onset diabetes is due to overweight. Physical exercise and fitness improves glucose tolerance without a change in body weight.
- Exercise in the form of walking can reduce the frequency of headaches and help the body to dissolve blood clots, as well as preventing varicose veins.
- Walking for 45–60 minutes twice a week can relieve depression and feelings of hopelessness.

So something which is as natural as breathing can have enormous benefits for total health. When you walk you use nearly *all* the muscles in your body, and the chances of stress and strain on bones and joints are greatly reduced. Moreover, it is a form of exercise you can do anywhere and at any time.

Your goal should be to walk at four miles per hour – a mile in 15 minutes – but you must build up to this slowly. Start by walking one to three miles at a slow pace, then after a week or two walk the same distance at a moderate pace. Several weeks later you should find it easy to walk a mile in 15 minutes. To help you assess your speed of walking, 120 steps a minute is approximately three and a half miles to the hour. This type of walking will give you aerobic-type exercise with your pulse reaching 70–85% of maximum capacity. To find your maximum capacity, subtract your age from 220 and 70–85% of this figure is the pulse rate you should aim for when walking. If you have never taken your own pulse, now is the time to learn. Place the tips of two fingers of one hand just below the thumb on the inside of the wrist of your other hand. Apply light pressure and you will feel the beat. Count your pulse for ten seconds by using a watch with a second hand, then multiply by six. (*Don't* use your thumb to take your pulse, as it has a pulse of its own.)

You must never overdo exercise. When walking you should be able to talk to a friend as you go along, never feel any pain and not be excessively tired when you've finished.

In the early stages you might like to do this breathing exercise, which will strengthen your heart and lungs and ensure you take in plenty of oxygen. Remember to stop as soon as you feel tired.

Take in a slow deep breath as you walk three paces, hold it for the next three paces, then let the breath out slowly with the last three paces. As you get used to this exercise, you can increase the steps following the same routine:

    slow intake of breath – over four paces
    hold breath   – for four paces
    breathe out slowly   – over four paces.

Do this when you're walking up a slope or hill and you will know you're exercising!

The advice I've given is not intended to stop you from taking any form of exercise you wish, but to point out that a very simple form of exercise – walking – has tremendous benefits for health and you are unlikely to do yourself any harm. Aim to make exercise – plus the relaxation method of your choice – a daily routine and the benefits will be obvious fairly quickly. Don't ever underestimate the effect stress has on the body. Drugs can never remove our problems; the most they can do is numb us over a period of time, only to have to face a stressful situation when the drug is no longer being taken. As I said in the nutritional chapter, a healthy way of eating can help the body cope with stress but cannot put right the root cause. So the conclusion has to be that we must help ourselves by facing up to difficulties, coping with them to the best of our ability and making sure we take time in our pressurized lives to relax. Relaxation is a great healer as well as an important preventive measure against poor future health.

CHAPTER ELEVEN

Case Histories

After going through the details of all the women seen at the Premenstrual Centre, I have picked out examples where a varied selection of remedies was taken. This shows that there is a choice available and it is a question of finding out what suits you. All were counselled on nutrition, and it is fair to say that those who followed the advice and changed their eating habits improved the most quickly. Many of the women seen were on drugs prescribed for PMT and were able to come off them with satisfactory results.

However, if you are taking drugs or under medical supervision, seek advice from your GP before embarking on any of the self-help cures mentioned in this book. Alternatively, if you think you are dependent on drugs, such as tranquillizers and sleeping pills, contact an organization specializing in drug abuse (*see* Chapter 12).

Case No. 1

Kathy, aged 26 with two children, had begun to experience PMT symptoms after the birth of her first child five years earlier. Fourteen days prior to her period, life was 'unbearable' due to severe fatigue, depression and mood changes. It was the lack of energy which bothered her the most and she was finding it difficult to cope with two young children. To a lesser extent she had discomfort from swollen breasts and gained up to five pounds before her period. Her doctor had prescribed a diuretic and had offered her tranquillizers which she had declined. Her weight had increased by fourteen pounds in the last year and she couldn't stick to a diet as she was always feeling hungry premenstrually.

She followed the nutritional advice and took Agnus Castus (herbal remedy) for her PMT symptoms, as well as following the three-hourly eating pattern for the last two weeks of her cycle.

After the first month all her symptoms except breast tenderness had gone, and she had an initial weight loss of six pounds. She continued with Agnus Castus and also added a Mega B time-release vitamin supplement. By the end of the second month she was entirely recovered except for slight breast tenderness. Four months later I had a telephone call from Kathy to say that she was still following the nutritional advice, taking B vitamins and had stopped the Agnus Castus. The only symptom she now had was the breast tenderness four days prior to her period, during which time she took infusions of dandelion. The following month Kathy reported no further problems with fluid retention.

Case No. 2

Jane, aged 35, married with no children, recognized that her PMT symptoms had started two years previously. This had coincided with her starting to drink heavily in order to ease tension. She was under a lot of strain financially as she had just started up her own business. Long hours often meant skipping meals and eating her evening meal as late as 10.00 pm at night, when it was mainly convenience and take-away foods. Seven to ten days prior to her period she had difficulty in communicating, often lost her train of thought and was generally unsteady and shaky. Food cravings, especially for chocolate and alcohol, had also resulted in a weight problem.

I suggested Jane went to a specialist clinic for help for her alcohol problem. In conjunction with this I advised her to make sure that she was eating a sound, nutritionally balanced diet – keeping to a three-hourly eating pattern during the ten days prior to her period. Jane also paid attention to the need to relax and set aside two 15-minute periods during the day for overall relaxation. Efamol Evening Primrose oil (500 mg capsules) and Efavite (vitamin/mineral supplement) were taken as indicated daily. There was a marked improvement in the first month. By the end of the second month she felt 80% better and reduced the Efamol Evening Primrose oil to ten days prior to the period.

Case No. 3

This is an interesting case involving a simple change of nutrition. When Mary came to see me, she was feeling anxious as she was about to start a new job, and worried about her PMT symptoms which had been worsening over the last six months. Her main problems were water retention, fatigue and depression up to ten days before her period. She appeared to eat a very healthy diet, with lots of fresh fruit and vegetables. She kept a careful watch on dairy products and seldom ate chocolates, biscuits etc. However, nine months previously she had gone on holiday to Spain and returned with litres of olive oil, which she used liberally on her food and in cooking. Her favourite snacks were raw vegetables covered in olive oil with plenty of salt.

I suggested she substituted the olive oil with cold-pressed safflower oil, and reduced her salt intake, deleting it from her diet ten days before her period. After the first month, all her symptoms had gone.

Case No. 4

Lyn's symptoms had started four years previously at the age of thirty. They had been diagnosed by a doctor who had prescribed Cyclogest progesterone suppositories from day eleven to the start of her period. Although she said the suppositories had helped she was still very tired, her weight had increased ten pounds in a year and she had breast tenderness from day twenty. Her lack of energy was causing problems at work.

She decided to come off the suppositories and took Efamol Evening Primrose oil (500 mg) plus Efavite, three times a day after food all through the month. She refrained from all refined foods and followed the three-hourly eating pattern for two weeks prior to her period. One month later she felt 75% improvement; by the end of the third month she reported slight tiredness the day before her period, but other than that was symptom-free with a weight loss of six pounds. She stopped taking Evening Primrose oil and maintained her nutritional programme. No further symptoms were reported.

Case No. 5

Susan, 45, married with three children, had had PMT symptoms since the birth of her first child and they had become progressively worse as the years went by.

Originally her doctor had prescribed tranquillizers, but two years later refused to give her any more prescriptions. Her withdrawal symptoms were bad, so she went to a private doctor who prescribed more tranquillizers. For the past five years she had been visiting this doctor on a regular basis to get her supply of the drug, spending around £20 each time for the consultation plus prescription. I put her in touch with an organization which would be able to advise her where to go for help in coming off tranquillizers.

For her PMT symptoms Susan followed the nutritional plan, three-hourly eating pattern, and throughout the month took a Mega B time release vitamin supplement, along with chelated minerals, 1 × 200 IU Vitamin E and 500 g Vitamin C daily.

Every month showed a gradual improvement, but her progress was hindered due to the tranquillizer problem. Six months later she was off the drug – and had no PMT symptoms.

Case No. 6

Pamela, 23, worked in a boutique and was having to take 2–3 days off per month due to migraine-type attacks just prior to her period. Her other symptoms were fairly mild, including water retention, increased hunger and a bloated feeling.

She decided to concentrate on the nutritional advice, including the three-hourly eating plan. For her migraine-type attacks she chose to try Feverfew (homoeopathic remedy).

After the first month all Pamela's PMT symptoms were gone, except for the bad headache the day before her period. She continued with the Feverfew, and the second month passed without any further problems.

Case No. 7

Paula, aged 19, was a student at college, living with her parents and hoping to marry the following year. Her main problem was depression two days before her period, during which time she was easily reduced to tears. Her diet on the whole was well-balanced. Her intake of dairy products was high and she was advised on how to cope with this by changing to low-fat products. She took Sepia (homoeopathic remedy) for five days prior to her period and the depression and tearful episodes stopped.

CONCLUSION

Many women reported immediate relief by simply changing their diet and taking mineral and vitamin supplements. They found that once their bodies had stabilized, by watching their diet for the final 1–2 weeks of each month they were able to avoid PMT symptoms. However, a number reported that if they went back to their old eating habits the symptoms quickly returned. Although some women felt that a three-hourly eating pattern would be difficult to arrange, once they were organized and ate this way they found food cravings were no longer a problem. Also, many found they were losing their unwanted pounds without suffering hunger pangs or fatigue.

A large number of the women responded well with the use of Evening Primrose oil. In a number of cases where symptoms remained despite nutritional changes and taking the oil, Agnus Castus relieved the symptoms. Many women who chose to take this herbal remedy from the start reported that all symptoms had gone within 1–2 months. It appeared to be particularly effective for migraine-type headaches prior to the period. Homoeopathic remedies brought relief to many women with depression, tension and irritability symptoms.

Women who were on drugs or going through a stressful time in their lives had a more difficult task in reducing their PMT symptoms. Although their symptoms worsened prior to the period, some were present throughout the entire month. These women were advised to contact organizations which could help with their particular problems.

Finally, I repeat what I said at the beginning of this chapter – quickest to improve were the women who followed the nutritional advice. They were also able to keep their use of remedies to a minimum.

CHAPTER TWELVE

Useful Contacts

Having read this book, you may decide you need professional help. Listed here are various organizations which will be able to put you in touch with registered practitioners. *On no account go to anyone who is not registered with an association.* Other bodies mentioned can assist with alcohol, drugs and smoking addictions, also depression. If you want to learn more about the art of relaxation, I have listed organizations specializing in a number of different approaches. Lastly, if you have difficulties in finding certain remedies locally, you can order by mail through the companies mentioned at the end of the Directory.

For further advice on drug-free treatments for premenstrual tension:
The Basingstoke Clinic, 54/56 New Market Square, Basingstoke, Hampshire.
Tel: 0256 28128

Please enclose a stamped, addressed envelope with your queries.

HOMOEOPATHIC DOCTORS	*The Homoeopathic Development Foundation,* 19A Cavendish Square, London W1M 9AD Tel: 01-629 3205 Monday–Friday, 10.00 am–4.30 pm.
	Australian Homeopathic Society, c/o Post Office, Darling Street Rozelle, NSW 2039

MEDICAL HERBALISTS	*The National Institute of Medical Herbalists,* Herbal Treatment Centre, 41 Hatherley Road, Winchester, Hampshire. Tel: Mrs Janet Hicks, MNIMH, on 0962 68776 *The National Herbalist Association of Australia* 49 Oakwood Street, Sutherland, NSW 2232
NATUROPATHS AND OSTEOPATHS	*British Naturopathic and Osteopathic Association,* Frazer House, 6 Netherhall Gardens, London NW3 5RR Tel: 01-435 7830
ACUPUNCTURISTS	*British Acupuncture Association and Register,* 34 Alderney Street, London SW1V 4EU Tel: 01-834 3353/1012 *Acupuncture Association of Australia* 1 Palmer Street, North Parramatta, NSW 2151
ALCOHOL ADDICTION	*Accept,* 200 Seagrave Road, London SW6 Tel: 01-381 3155 *Alcoholics Anonymous,* Box 514, 11 Redcliffe Gardens, London SW10 Tel: 01-352 9779

Westminster Advisory Centre on Alcoholism,
38 Ebury Street,
London SW1W 0LU
Tel: 01-730 1574

Alcoholics Anonymous,
363 George Street,
Sydney, NSW 2000

DRUG ADDICTION

Release,
Tel: 01-603 8654
Although this organization specializes in the area of illegal drug abuse, it can assist with initial advice and information on tranquillizer addiction.

Standing Conference on Drug Abuse (SCODA),
1–4 Hatton Place,
London EC1N 8ND
Tel: 01-430 2341
A voluntary organization co-ordinating information nationwide on drug abuse. (This does not include alcohol and nicotine addiction.)

Centre for Education and Information on Drugs and Alcohol,
Dowling Street,
Surrey Hills, NSW 2010

SMOKING

ASH (Action on Smoking and Health),
5–11 Mortimer Street,
London W1
Tel: 01-637 9843

Anti-Cancer Council of NSW,
10 Martin Place,
Sydney, NSW 2000

DEPRESSION

Samaritans,
17 Uxbridge Road, Slough, Berkshire
Tel: Slough 32713/4
Counselling for the depressed, despairing
and suicidal. Local branch addresses in
your phone book.

Samaritans (Australia),
60 Bagot Road,
Subiaco, Perth, WA 6008

RELAXATION

British Wheel of Yoga,
General Secretary, 80 Lechampton Road,
Cheltenham, Glos.
They have a list of qualified teachers
throughout the country. Also contact
your local education authority.

International Institute of Reflexology,
PO Box 34, Harlow, Essex CM17 0LT
Lists of qualified therapists throughout
UK and Europe available.

Shiatsu Society,
188 Old Street,
London EC1
Tel: 01-278 6783
Holds a list of practitioners and teachers
in the UK.

*Society of Teachers of the Alexander
Technique,*
10 London House, 266 Fulham Road,
London SW10
Tel: 01-584 3834
The Society holds a directory of all
recognized teachers in the UK.

Touch for Health Foundation,
39 Browns Road, Surbiton, Surrey
Tel: 01-399 3215
Provides training courses and has a list of
instructors throughout the UK. It is also
an applied kinesiology clinic.

HOMOEOPATHIC REMEDIES

A. Nelson & Co. Ltd.,
5 Endeavour Way,
Wimbledon SW19 9UH
Tel: 01-946 8527

Weleda (UK) Ltd.,
Heanor Road, Ilkeston, Derbyshire
DE7 8DR
Tel: 0602 303151

Both these companies offer a mail order
service.

DRIED HERBS

Culpeper Ltd.,
Hadstock Road, Linton, Cambridge
CB1 6NJ
Tel: 0223 891196

Gerard House (1965) Ltd.,
736b Christchurch Road, Boscombe,
Bournemouth, Dorset
Tel: 0202 35352

Neals Yard Apothecary,
No. 2 Neals Yard, Covent Garden,
London WC2
Tel: 01-379 7222

All the above companies offer a mail
order service.

LOCAL SHOPPING FOR REMEDIES AND SUPPLEMENTS
Vitamins, minerals and other dietary supplements mentioned in
this book can be purchased at health food shops, which also stock

homoeopathic remedies and herbal tablets. Dietary supplements are also available at chemists'. Homoeopathic remedies and herbal preparations are starting to appear on some chemists' shelves, so it's worth having a look. If you cannot find what you are looking for, ask if they will order. Chemists are more likely to stock remedies if they feel there is public demand.

CHAPTER THIRTEEN

Summary Charts

TYPE 1	*Depression, confusion, lack of concentration, clumsiness*
NUTRITION	Follow the general nutritional advice throughout the month. Three-hourly eating plan during PMT phase.
VITAMINS & MINERALS	B complex *or* a combination of B1, B2 and B6. Chelated minerals with particular attention to magnesium and zinc.
DIETARY SUPPLEMENTS	Evening Primrose oil
HOMOEOPATHIC REMEDIES	Sepia, *Ignatia, Actea rac*.
HERBAL REMEDIES	Agnus Castus, Lemon Balm, Rosemary, St John's Wort
EXERCISE	Any form of moderate exercise
RELAXATION	Total Relaxation Routine
ACUPRESSURE POINTS	Exercise 5

TYPE 2	*Tension: irritability, aggression, mood changes, anxiety*
NUTRITION	Follow the general nutritional advice throughout the month. Three-hourly eating plan during PMT phase.
VITAMINS & MINERALS	B Complex or a combination of B1, B2 and B6, plus Vitamin C. Chelated minerals with particular attention to Magnesium and Zinc.
DIETARY SUPPLEMENTS	Evening Primrose oil
HOMOEOPATHIC REMEDIES	Sulphur, *Nux vom., Bryonia, Arsen. alb., Argent. nit., Apis mel., Aconite.*
HERBAL REMEDIES	Agnus Castus, Lemon Balm, Motherwort, Sage Leaves, Valerian
EXERCISE	Any form of moderate exercise
RELAXATION	Total Relaxation Routine
ACUPRESSURE POINTS	Exercises 4 and 5

TYPE 3	*Water retention: sore breasts, weight gain, bloatedness*
NUTRITION	Follow the general nutritional advice throughout the month. Avoid any form of salt during PMT phase, and reduce saturated fats.
VITAMINS & MINERALS	B Complex and chelated minerals paying particular attention to Vitamin C, Vitamin E, Magnesium and Potassium.
DIETARY SUPPLEMENTS	Evening Primrose oil
HOMOEOPATHIC REMEDIES	*Calc. carb., Lachesis*
HERBAL REMEDIES	Agnus Castus, Dandelion Leaf, Couch Grass, Vervain
EXERCISE	Any form of moderate exercise

TYPE 4	*Food cravings: sugar and carbohydrate cravings, headaches, fatigue* NB As there are many types of headache all remedies and acupressure points for headaches are shown in brackets. You should refer to the chapters concerned and choose remedies and/or exercises that match your symptoms.
NUTRITION	Follow the general nutritional advice throughout the month. During PMT phase avoid alcohol and all products containing sugar and refined carbohydrates. Go on the three hourly eating plan.
VITAMINS & MINERALS	B Complex and Vitamin E. Chelated minerals, particularly Magnesium and Potassium
DIETARY SUPPLEMENTS	Lejguar guar gum
HOMOEOPATHIC REMEDIES	*Pulsatilla, Lycopodium,* Graphites, *Ferr. phos., Calc. carb.,* (*Silicea, Nat. mur., Kali. phos., Kali. bich., Ignatia, Euphrasia,* Feverfew)
HERBAL REMEDIES	(Feverfew, Vervain, Valerian, Rosemary, Meadowsweet, Lavender, Catmint)
EXERCISE	Any form of moderate exercise
RELAXATION	Total Relaxation Routine
ACUPRESSURE POINTS	Exercises 6 and 7 (1, 2 and 3)

Reading Material

Clinical Uses of Essential Fatty Acids Ed. David F. Horrobin (Eden Press, 1983)

Complete Guide to Prescription and Non-Prescription Drugs H. Winter Griffith MD (HP Books, 1983)

Cured to Death Arabella Melville and Colin Johnson (New English Library, 1983)

Green Pharmacy Barbara Griggs (Jill Norman & Hobhouse, 1981)

The Homoeopathic Handbook Ed. T. M. Cole (Nelson, 1980)

Let's Get Well Adelle Davis (Unwin Paperbacks, 1979)

Raw Energy Leslie Kenton (Century, 1984)

Low Blood Sugar (Hypoglycaemia) – The Twentieth-Century Epidemic? Martin L. Budd ND, DO, Lic.Ac. (Thorsons, 1981)

No More Menstrual Cramps and Other Good News Dr Penny Wise Budoff MD (Angus & Robertson, 1984)

Once a Month Dr Katharina Dalton (Harvester Press, 1979; Fontana, 1983)

The Aromatherapy Handbook Daniele Ryman (Century, 1984)

onthly Chart

Nov '86

NTH:

k Your Symptoms as Follows: ☐ None ◲ Mild ⊠ Moderate ■ Severe

																		P	P	P P											
TYPE	**PMT SYMPTOMS**	1	2	3	4	5	6	7	8	9	10	11	12	13	14	15	16	17	18	19	20	21	22	23	24	25	26	27	28	29	30	31
	Depression																															
	Weepiness																		⊠	⊠												
	Lack of concentration																															
	Lack of sleep														⊠	⊠																
	Clumsiness																															
	Tension																															
	Aggression					⊠								⊠	⊠	⊠																
	Mood changes																															
	Anxiety																															
	Irritability																															
	Sore breasts																															
	Weight gain																															
	Swollen joints																															
	Bloating																															
	Food cravings																		⊠													
	Headaches																				⊠											
	Fatigue																⊠	⊠	⊠													
	Alcohol craving																															
	Lack of sex drive																															
	Skin problems																															
	Backache																															
	Hot flushes																															

Personal Notes

H:

Your Symptoms as Follows: ☐ None ▨ Mild ⊠ Moderate ■ Severe

PMT SYMPTOMS	DAYS OF THE MONTH																														
	1	2	3	4	5	6	7	8	9	10	11	12	13	14	15	16	17	18	19	20	21	22	23	24	25	26	27	28	29	30	31
Depression																															
Weepiness																															
Lack of concentration																															
Lack of sleep																															
Clumsiness																															
Tension																															
Aggression																															
Mood changes																															
Anxiety																															
Irritability																															
Sore breasts																															
Weight gain																															
Swollen joints																															
Bloating																															
Food cravings																															
Headaches																															
Fatigue																															
Alcohol craving																															
Lack of sex drive																															
Skin problems																															
Backache																															
Hot flushes																															

Personal Notes

Monthly Chart

MONTH:

Mark Your Symptoms as Follows: ☐ None ◩ Mild ⊠ Moderate ■ Severe

TYPE	PMT SYMPTOMS	\multicolumn{31}{c}{DAYS OF THE MONTH}																															
		1	2	3	4	5	6	7	8	9	10	11	12	13	14	15	16	17	18	19	20	21	22	23	24	25	26	27	28	29	30	31
1	Depression																															
	Weepiness																															
	Lack of concentration																															
	Lack of sleep																															
	Clumsiness																															
2	Tension																															
	Aggression																															
	Mood changes																															
	Anxiety																															
	Irritability																															
3	Sore breasts																															
	Weight gain																															
	Swollen joints																															
	Bloating																															
4	Food cravings																															
	Headaches																															
	Fatigue																															
	Alcohol craving																															
MISC	Lack of sex drive																															
	Skin problems																															
	Backache																															
	Hot flushes																															

Personal Notes

onthly Chart

ark Your Symptoms as Follows: ☐ None ◻ Mild ⊠ Moderate ■ Severe

		DAYS OF THE MONTH																														
YPE	PMT SYMPTOMS	1	2	3	4	5	6	7	8	9	10	11	12	13	14	15	16	17	18	19	20	21	22	23	24	25	26	27	28	29	30	31
1	Depression																															
	Weepiness																															
	Lack of concentration																															
	Lack of sleep																															
	Clumsiness																															
2	Tension																															
	Aggression																															
	Mood changes																															
	Anxiety																															
	Irritability																															
3	Sore breasts																															
	Weight gain																															
	Swollen joints																															
	Bloating																															
4	Food cravings																															
	Headaches																															
	Fatigue																															
	Alcohol craving																															
MISC	Lack of sex drive																															
	Skin problems																															
	Backache																															
	Hot flushes																															

Personal Notes

onthly Chart

NTH:

rk Your Symptoms as Follows: ☐ None ☐ Mild ☒ Moderate ■ Severe

PE	PMT SYMPTOMS	DAYS OF THE MONTH																													
		1	2	3	4	5	6	7	8	9	10	11	12	13	14	15	16	17	18	19	20	21	22	23	24	25	26	27	28	29	30	31
₁	Depression																																
	Weepiness																																
	Lack of concentration																																
	Lack of sleep																																
	Clumsiness																																
₂	Tension																																
	Aggression																																
	Mood changes																																
	Anxiety																																
	Irritability																																
₃	Sore breasts																																
	Weight gain																																
	Swollen joints																																
	Bloating																																
₄	Food cravings																																
	Headaches																																
	Fatigue																																
	Alcohol craving																																
M ₅ C	Lack of sex drive																																
	Skin problems																																
	Backache																																
	Hot flushes																																

Personal Notes

onthly Chart

MONTH:

Mark Your Symptoms as Follows: ☐ None ◨ Mild ⊠ Moderate ■ Severe

TYPE	PMT SYMPTOMS	DAYS OF THE MONTH																														
		1	2	3	4	5	6	7	8	9	10	11	12	13	14	15	16	17	18	19	20	21	22	23	24	25	26	27	28	29	30	31
1	Depression																															
	Weepiness																															
	Lack of concentration																															
	Lack of sleep																															
	Clumsiness																															
2	Tension																															
	Aggression																															
	Mood changes																															
	Anxiety																															
	Irritability																															
3	Sore breasts																															
	Weight gain																															
	Swollen joints																															
	Bloating																															
4	Food cravings																															
	Headaches																															
	Fatigue																															
	Alcohol craving																															
MISC	Lack of sex drive																															
	Skin problems																															
	Backache																															
	Hot flushes																															

Personal Notes

Index

acupressure 99–103
acupuncture xii, 99
additives 23, 29
adrenal glands 12, 28
adrenalin 12
Agnus Castus 82–3, 109, 112
alcohol 6, 8, 18, 29, 36, 109
alcoholism 15, 115
Alexander principle 104
applied kinesiology 104
aromatic oils 104
arthritis 23
artificial sweeteners 29
aspirin 82

balanced diet 25
biotin 8
blood sugar levels 11
bran 43
breathing exercise 107
Brewer's yeast 31
Budoff, Penny Wise 4

caffeine 29
cancer 23

carbohydrates 23, 25, 26, 44, 46
carotene 27
cis-linoleic acid 6–8
coffee 16, 18, 20, 29, 32
contraceptive pill 16, 50, 51, 52, 53, 54, 56
cooking tips 30
corpus luteum 3
cortisone 12
crime 15

Dalton, Dr Katharina 3–5, 123
decoctions 83
depression x–xii, 1, 11, 12, 24, 56, 63, 66, 78–9, 86, 90, 106, 112, 116, 119
diabetes 6, 12, 23, 43, 106
drugs ix, 1, 4, 24, 53, 108, 111

emotional sickness 24
endometrium 2
essential amino acids 27
essential fatty acids (EFAs) 5, 25

Evening Primrose oil 6–8, 57–8, 109–10, 112
exercise 105–7

fasting blood-sugar test 13
fatigue x–xii, 1, 11, 24, 49, 91, 96, 108
fats 25–6
fibre, sources of 43–6
follicle stimulating hormone 3
food industry 23
fructose 27

gammalinolenic acid (GLA) 5–8, 57–8
guar gum 45–6
Gwinup, Dr Grant 105–6

Hahnemann, Dr Samuel 59–60
Harris, Dr Seale 11
herbal remedies 16, 81–9, 117–18; *for*: depression 86; fluid retention 84; general health tonics 87; headache 85; heavy periods 88; insomnia 86; irregular periods 89; migraine 86; painful periods 88; scanty periods 89; sickness and nausea 87; tension 87
herbalism 81
Hibiscus rosa sinensis 82
homoeopathic medicines 16, 59–80, 117; *for*: anxiety 63; breast tenderness 63; confusion 63; depression 63; excess fat 64; excessive appetite 63; headaches 64; irritability 64; migraine 65; sugar/carbohydrate cravings 65
hormone levels xii, 1, 3, 4
hypoglycaemia xii, 11–14, 23, 57, 123
hypothalmus 3

infusions 83, 109
insulin 8, 12, 27

kelp 28, 31

lecithin 31
linoleic acid 5, 7
linseed 31
lutenising hormone 3
low blood sugar 11–13, 123

margarine 19, 26
massage 104
menus, daily 32–3
minerals 25, 55–8; calcium 27, 55; chelated 48; magnesium 6, 8, 56, 58; potassium 27, 56–7; zinc 6, 8, 57–8
monthly cycle 2–3

nutrition 18–41, 109, 110, 111, 112, 113
nutritionist 25

oestrogen 3, 4, 9, 57
organic hypoglycaemia 12–13

pectin 44
pituitary gland 3, 5, 12
potassium-sodium balance 28
progesterone x, xi, 3, 4, 5, 9;
    injections 4; suppositories 4,
    110; versus placebo
    research 5
prolactin 5, 9
prostaglandin E1 7–10
protein 27
pulse rate 107

radioimmunoassay 4
Randolph, Dr Theroux G. 48
reactive hypoglycaemia
    12–13
recipes 37–41; Baked Fish 39;
    Crunchy Raw Salad 38;
    Healthy Dessert 41; Lentil
    Shepherd's Pie 41; Modified
    Butter 37; Salad Dressing
    37; Spinach Open Omelette
    40; Vegetable Soup 37;
    Yoghurt and Tomato Juice
    Cocktail 38
reflexology 104
relaxation 96–105, 109, 116–
    17
relaxation routine 97–99

salt 19, 28, 110
Sampson, Dr Gwyneth 5
saturated fats 23, 25, 29, 57

shiatsu 104
shopping list, basic 30
six-hour glucose tolerance test
    11, 13
soluble fibre 43–5
sprouting seeds 28
starches 26
stress 11, 16, 51, 53, 56, 90–
    95; check list 92–3; coping
    strategies profile 94–5; and
    the menstrual cycle 91;
    symptoms of 90
sugar 19, 23, 26, 27, 29; and
    carbohydrate cravings ix,
    xii, 1, 34–7, 42, 65, 75,
    109, 122
suicide x, 11, 15

tea 29
thyroid gland xii, 12
trans-linoleic acid 5–7

unsaturated fats 25–6

vitamins 25, 47–54; A 50, 54,
    57; B complex 8, 49, 109;
    B1 50–1; B2 51; B6 6, 8,
    52, 57, 58; C 8, 27, 48, 50,
    52–3, 54; E 6, 50, 54; F 26;
    time release 48

walking 105–7
water retention 15, 42–3, 51,
    52, 54, 64, 84, 108, 110,
    121

wheatgerm 31, 57
wholefood shops 23
willow (*salix alba*) 81

yoga 101

Zoapatl (*Montanor tormentosa*) 82

Notes

Notes

Notes